Endoscopy and Liver Disease

Guest Editors

ANDRÉS CÁRDENAS, MD, MMSc
PAUL J. THULUVATH, MD, FRCP

CLINICS IN LIVER DISEASE

www.liver.theclinics.com

Consulting Editor
NORMAN M. GITLIN, MD

May 2010 • Volume 14 • Number 2

SAUNDERS an imprint of ELSEVIER, Inc.

W.B. SAUNDERS COMPANY

A Division of Elsevier Inc.

1600 John F. Kennedy Boulevard, Suite 1800 • Philadelphia, PA 19103-2899

http://www.theclinics.com

CLINICS IN LIVER DISEASE Volume 14, Number 2
May 2010 ISSN 1089-3261, ISBN-13: 978-1-4377-1914-7

Editor: Kerry Holland

Clinics in Liver Disease (ISSN 1089-3261) is published quarterly by Elsevier Inc., 360 Park Avenue South, New York, NY 10010-1710. Months of issue are February, May, August, and November. Business and Editorial Offices: 1600 John F. Kennedy Blvd., Ste. 1800, Philadelphia, PA 19103-2899. Customer Service Office: 3251 Riverport Lane, Maryland Heights, MO 63043. Periodicals postage paid at New York, NY and additional mailing offices. Subscription prices are $235.00 per year (U.S. individuals), $118.00 per year (U.S. student/resident), $340.00 per year (U.S. institutions), $311.00 per year (foreign individuals), $163.00 per year (foreign student/ resident), $409.00 per year (foreign instituitions), $271.00 per year (Canadian individuals), $163.00 per year (Canadian student/resident), and $409.00 per year (Canadian institutions). Foreign air speed delivery is included in all *Clinics* subscription prices. All prices are subject to change without notice. **POSTMASTER:** Send address changes to *Clinics in Liver Disease*, Elsevier Health Sciences Division, Subscription Customer Service, 3251 Riverport Lane, Maryland Heights, MO 63043. **Customer Service: Telephone: 1-800-654-2452 (U.S. and Canada); 314-447-8871 (outside U.S. and Canada). Fax: 314-447-8029. E-mail: journalscustomer service-usa@elsevier.com (for print support); journalsonlinesupport-usa@elsevier.com (for online support).**

Reprints. For copies of 100 or more of articles in this publication, please contact the Commercial Reprints Department, Elsevier Inc., 360 Park Avenue South, New York, NY 10010-1710. Tel.: 212-633-3812; Fax: 212-462-1935; E-mail: reprints@elsevier.com.

Clinics in Liver Disease is covered in *MEDLINE/PubMed (Index Medicus)*.

Printed and bound by CPI Group (UK) Ltd, Croydon, CR0 4YY

Transferred to Digital Print 2011

Contributors

CONSULTING EDITOR

NORMAN M. GITLIN, MD, FRCP(London), FRCPE(Edinburgh), FACG, FACP
Formerly, Professor of Medicine, Chief of Hepatology, Emory University; Currently, Consultant, Atlanta Gastroenterology Associates, Atlanta, Georgia

GUEST EDITORS

ANDRÉS CÁRDENAS, MD, MMSc
Faculty Member GI Unit / Institut Clinic de Malalties Digestives i Metaboliques, University of Barcelona, Hospital Clinic, Barcelona, Spain

PAUL J. THULUVATH, MD, FRCP
Professor of Surgery and Medicine, Georgetown University School of Medicine; Medical Director, Institute for Digestive Health and Liver Diseases, Mercy Medical Center, Baltimore, Maryland

AUTHORS

AGUSTÍN ALBILLOS, MD, PhD
Professor of Medicine, Servicio de Gastroenterología y Hepatología, Hospital Universitario Ramón y Cajal, Universidad de Alcalá; Centro de Investigación Biomédica en Red de Enfermedades Hepáticas y Digestivas (Ciberehd), Instituto de Salud Carlos III, Madrid, Spain

NEVILLE BAMJI, MD
Clinical Instructor, Division of Gastroenterology, Department of Medicine, Mount Sinai School of Medicine, New York, New York

TODD H. BARON, MD, FASGE
Professor of Medicine, Division of Gastroenterology and Hepatology, Mayo Clinic Rochester, Rochester, Minnesota

ANNALISA BERZIGOTTI, MD, PhD
Research Fellow, Hepatic Hemodynamic Laboratory, Liver Unit, Hospital Clinic, Institut d'Investigacions Biomediques August Pi i Sunyer (IDIBAPS) and Centro de Investigación Biomédica en Red de Enfermedades Hepáticas y Digestivas (CIBERehd); Specialist, Ultrasound Unit, Centre de Diagnostic por la Imatge (CDIC), Hospital Clinic, University of Barcelona, Barcelona, Spain

ANDRÉS CÁRDENAS, MD, MMSc
Faculty Member GI Unit / Institut Clinic de Malalties Digestives i Metaboliques, University of Barcelona, Hospital Clinic, Barcelona, Spain

NAYANTARA COELHO-PRABHU, MD
Fellow, Division of Gastroenterology and Hepatology, Mayo Clinic Rochester, Rochester, Minnesota

LAWRENCE B. COHEN, MD
Associate Clinical Professor, Division of Gastroenterology, Department of Medicine, Mount Sinai School of Medicine, New York, New York

MARIO D'AMICO, MD
Research Fellow, Hepatic Hemodynamic Laboratory, Liver Unit, Hospital Clinic, Institut d'Investigacions Biomediques August Pi i Sunyer (IDIBAPS) and Centro de Investigación Biomédica en Red de Enfermedades Hepáticas y Digestivas (CIBERehd), University of Barcelona, Barcelona, Spain

ROBERTO DE FRANCHIS, MD
Università degli Studi di Milano, IRCCS Ca' Granda Ospedale Policlinico Foundation, Gastroenterologia 3, Milano, Italy

ALESSANDRA DELL' ERA, MD, PhD
Università degli Studi di Milano, IRCCS Ca' Granda Ospedale Policlinico Foundation, Gastroenterologia 3, Milano, Italy

GLÒRIA FERNÁNDEZ-ESPARRACH, MD, PhD
Endoscopy Unit, Institut de Malalties Digestives i Metabòliques, Hospital Clínic, CIBERehd, IDIBAPS, University of Barcelona, Barcelona, Spain

JUAN CARLOS GARCIA-PAGAN, MD, PhD
Senior Consultant, Hepatic Hemodynamic Laboratory, Liver Unit, Hospital Clinic, Institut d'Investigacions Biomediques August Pi i Sunyer (IDIBAPS) and Centro de Investigación Biomédica en Red de Enfermedades Hepáticas y Digestivas (CIBERehd), University of Barcelona, Barcelona, Spain

GUADALUPE GARCIA-TSAO, MD
Professor of Medicine, Section of Digestive Diseases, Yale University School of Medicine and VA-CT Healthcare System, New Haven, Connecticut

ANGELS GINÈS, MD, PhD
Endoscopy Unit, Institut de Malalties Digestives i Metabòliques, Hospital Clínic, CIBERehd, IDIBAPS, University of Barcelona, Barcelona, Spain

DANIEL GOTTHARDT, MD
Department of Medicine, Medizinische Universitätsklinik, University of Heidelberg, Heidelberg, Germany

SANJAY JAGANNATH, MD
Institute for Digestive Health and Liver Diseases, Mercy Medical Center, Baltimore, Maryland

PATRICK S. KAMATH, MD
Professor of Medicine, Division of Gastroenterology and Hepatology, Mayo Clinic Rochester, Rochester, Minnesota

SERGEY KANTSEVOY, MD, PhD
Institute for Digestive Health and Liver Diseases, Mercy Medical Center, Baltimore, Maryland

KAREN L. KROK, MD
Assistant Professor of Medicine, Division of Gastroenterology, University of Pennsylvania School of Medicine, Philadelphia, Pennsylvania

GIN-HO LO, MD
Director, Department of Medical Education, Digestive Center, E-DA Hospital, Kaohsiung County; Professor, I-Shou University, Kaohsiung, Taiwan, Republic of China

ANURAG MAHESHWARI, MD
Institute for Digestive Health and Liver Diseases, Mercy Medical Center, Baltimore, Maryland

S.R. MISHRA, MD, DM
Department of Gastroenterology, G B Pant Hospital, New Delhi, India

BEATRIZ PEÑAS, MD
Servicio de Gastroenterología y Hepatología, Hospital Universitario Ramón y Cajal, Universidad de Alcalá, Madrid, Spain

CRISTINA RIPOLL, MD
Attending Physician, Hepatology and Liver Transplant Unit, Department of Digestive Diseases, Hospital General Universitario Gregorio Marañón, Madrid, Spain

EMANUELE RONDONOTTI, MD, PhD
Universitàdegli Studi di Milano, IRCCS Ca' Granda Ospedale Policlinico Foundation, Gastroenterologia 3, Milano, Italy

S.K. SARIN, MD, DM
Department of Gastroenterology, G B Pant Hospital, University of Delhi, and Project Director, Institute of Liver and Biliary Sciences (ILBS), New Delhi, India

ADOLF STIEHL, MD
Professor of Medicine, Department of Medicine, Medizinische Universitätsklinik, University of Heidelberg, Heidelberg, Germany

PAUL J. THULUVATH, MD, FRCP
Professor of Surgery and Medicine, Georgetown University School of Medicine; Medical Director, Institute for Digestive Health and Liver Diseases, Mercy Medical Center, Baltimore, Maryland

GIAN EUGENIO TONTINI, MD
Università degli Studi di Milano, IRCCS Ca' Granda Ospedale Policlinico Foundation, Gastroenterologia 3, Milano, Italy

FEDERICA VILLA, MD
Università degli Studi di Milano IRCCS Ca' Granda Ospedale Policlinico Foundation, Gastroenterologia 3, Milano, Italy

JAVIER ZAMORA, MD, PhD
Servicio de Bioestadística Clínica, Hospital Universitario Ramón y Cajal, Universidad de Alcalá; Centro de Investigación Biomédica en Red Epidemiología y Salud Pública (Ciberesp), Instituto de Salud Carlos III, Madrid, Spain

Contents

Preface **xiii**

Andrés Cárdenas and Paul J. Thuluvath

Endoscopic Sedation of Patients with Chronic Liver Disease **185**

Neville Bamji and Lawrence B. Cohen

Endoscopic procedures are often necessary in patients with chronic liver disease. The preprocedure evaluation of such patients should include an assessment of hepatic synthetic function and identification of neuropsychiatric findings suggestive of hepatic encephalopathy. It may be possible, in some cases, to perform diagnostic esophagogastroduodenoscopy without administration of sedation; this is desirable to eliminate the risks of sedation, especially encephalopathy. Nonetheless, most patients undergoing upper and lower endoscopy require sedation. Currently, the use of propofol is preferred to benzodiazepines and opioids for endoscopic sedation of patients with advanced liver disease due to its short biologic half-life and low risk of provoking hepatic encephalopathy. In appropriately selected patients, gastroenterologist-directed propofol administration seems safe.

Current Staging and Diagnosis of Gastroesophageal Varices **195**

Nayantara Coelho-Prabhu and Patrick S. Kamath

Portal hypertension is defined as an increase in hepatic sinusoidal pressure to 6 mm Hg or higher. Cirrhosis is the most common cause of portal hypertension in the western world and results from increased resistance to blood flow at the hepatic sinusoidal level.

Capsule Endoscopy in Portal Hypertension **209**

Emanuele Rondonotti, Federica Villa, Alessandra Dell' Era, Gian Eugenio Tontini, and Roberto de Franchis

Since the introduction of small bowel capsule endoscopy, and more recently of esophageal capsule endoscopy, these diagnostic tools have become available for the evaluation of the consequences of portal hypertension in the esophagus, stomach, and small intestine. The main advantage of the esophageal and the small bowel capsule is the relatively less invasiveness that could potentially increase patients' adherence to endoscopic screening/surveillance programs. When esophageal capsule endoscopy was compared with traditional gastroscopy, it showed good sensitivity and specificity in recognizing the presence and the size of esophageal varices. However, the results are not consistent among studies, and more data are needed.

FORTHCOMING ISSUES

August 2010
Hepatitis B Virus
Naoky Tsai, MD, *Guest Editor*

November 2010
Liver Pathology
Jay H. Lefkowitch, MD, *Guest Editor*

February 2011
Hepatic Manifestations of Systemic Disease
Ke-Qin Hu, MD, *Guest Editor*

RECENT ISSUES

February 2010
Health Care-Associated Transmission of Hepatitis B and C Viruses
Bandar Al Knawy, MD, FRCPC, *Guest Editor*

November 2009
Non-Alcoholic Steatohepatitis
Stephen A. Harrison, MD, LTC, MC, FACP, *Guest Editor*

August 2009
Novel Therapies in Hepatitis C Virus
Paul J. Pockros, MD, *Guest Editor*

RELATED INTEREST

Gastrointestinal Endoscopy Clinics of North America, October 2009, Vol. 19, No. 4
Intraductal Biliary and Pancreatic Endoscopy
Peter D. Stevens, MD, *Guest Editor*

Preface

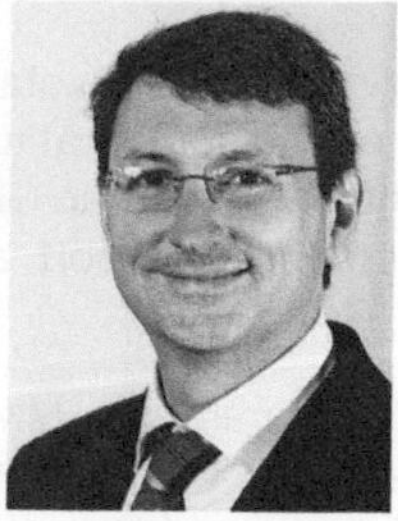

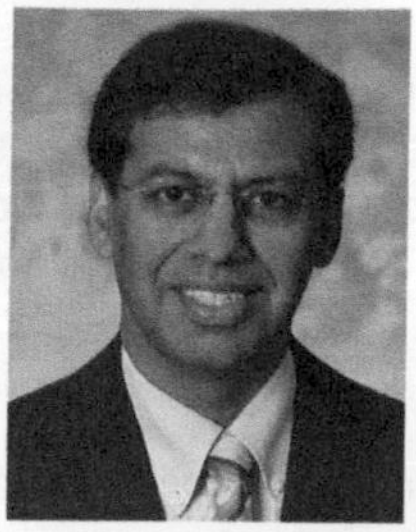

Andrés Cárdenas, MD, MMSc Paul J. Thuluvath, MD, FRCP
Guest Editors

The field of hepatology has advanced enormously in the past two decades. Novel diagnostic and therapeutic interventions in clinical hepatology and liver transplantation have grown exponentially during this period, and subspecialty interests have emerged within the liver disease arena. Endoscopy plays an important role in the management of patients of hepatobiliary diseases, yet it has remained in the periphery of this specialty. We believe that a better understanding of the indications, the diagnostic and therapeutic possibilities, the limitations, and the potential complications of endoscopic interventions are essential for those who manage patients with chronic hepatobiliary diseases and liver transplantation. In this issue, we have assembled an outstanding group of experts in the field of endoscopy and hepatology who share their vast experience and critically appraise important endoscopic developments in the management of patients with hepatobiliary diseases.

The optimal sedation of patients with liver disease undergoing endoscopic procedures is poorly defined, and this issue starts with a detailed discussion of this topic by Drs Bamjii and Cohen. In the second article, Drs Coelho-Prabhu and Kamath appraise the current staging methods and the various diagnostic modalities for gastroesophageal varices. This is followed by a detailed analysis of the role of capsule endoscopy in patients with portal hypertension by Dr deFranchis and colleagues. Endoscopic ultrasound may play an important role in the diagnosis of portal hypertension and liver masses, and these topics are reviewed by Drs Gines and Thuluvath, respectively. The role of endoscopy for primary and secondary prophylaxis of gastroesophageal varices is discussed by Drs Albillos and Lo, respectively. Acute variceal bleeding is a medical emergency where optimal treatment is often life saving. The management is complex and may involve endoscopic, pharmacologic, and nonendoscopic interventions. These topics are reviewed in detail by Dr Cardenas and by D'Amico and colleagues. The current management of gastric varices, portal hypertensive gastropathy, and gastric antral vascular ectasia and gastric varices is discussed by Drs Sarin and coworkers and by Drs Ripoll and Garcia-Tsao. Endoscopic retrograde cholangiopancreatography (ERCP) continues to be the diagnostic and therapeutic procedure of choice for patients with primary sclerosing cholangitis and extrahepatic

Clin Liver Dis 14 (2010) xiii–xiv
doi:10.1016/j.cld.2010.04.001

cholangiocarcinoma. The role of ERCP in PSC is evaluated by Drs Gotthardt and Stiehl and its role in cholangiocarcinoma by Drs Coelho-Prabhu and Baron. Lastly, we critically appraise the role of ERCP in the management of post–liver transplant biliary complications.

We sincerely hope that this issue has succeeded in summarizing the current status of endoscopy in the management of hepatobiliary diseases. We express our gratitude to all authors for their excellent contributions. Additionally, we thank Dr Norman Gitlin for entrusting us with this task and Kerry Holland for her editorial support and assistance.

Andrés Cárdenas, MD, MMSc
GI Unit / Institut Clinic de Malalties Digestives i Metaboliques
University of Barcelona
Hospital Clinic
Villarroel 170
Barcelona 08036, Spain

Paul J. Thuluvath, MD, FRCP
Georgetown University School of Medicine
Institute for Digestive Health and Liver Diseases Mercy Medical Center
Baltimore, MD 21202, USA

E-mail addresses:
acardena@clinic.ub.es (A. Cárdenas)
thuluvath@gmail.com (P.J. Thuluvath)

Endoscopic Sedation of Patients with Chronic Liver Disease

Neville Bamji, MD, Lawrence B. Cohen, MD*

KEYWORDS

- Chronic liver disease • Endoscopy • Sedation
- Minimal hepatic encephalopathy

Chronic diseases of the liver affect more than 5.5 million people in the United States.[1] Most of these individuals undergo an endoscopic examination at one time or another, whether or not it is a screening colonoscopy, a standard diagnostic endoscopy, or one performed to evaluate a complication of a patient's underlying liver disorder. Colonoscopy and esophagogastroduodenoscopy (EGD) are also routinely performed as part of a pretransplantation evaluation. Consequently, patients with chronic liver disease are likely to undergo 1 or more endoscopic examinations and, as discussed in this article, special consideration should be given to the method of sedation chosen for these patients. This article reviews the effects of chronic liver disease on the pharmacokinetic properties of commonly used sedation drugs and the sedation-related complications in chronic liver disease with particular focus on hepatic encephalopathy. The general principles of patient sedation and monitoring as well as recommendations for an approach to the sedation of patients with chronic liver disease are also provided.

HEPATIC DYSFUNCTION AND THE METABOLISM OF SEDATION DRUGS

Hepatic dysfunction as a result of liver disease can have a significant impact on drug metabolism and pharmacokinetics. These metabolic and physiologic derangements vary in severity, depending on the degree of hepatic dysfunction, and may include alterations in protein binding and reduced levels of serum albumin and other protein-binding proteins, changes in the volume of distribution due to ascites and increased total body water compartments, and slowed drug metabolism secondary to abnormal hepatocyte function.

Endoscopic sedation practices vary from country to country and sometimes between different regions of the same country. Within the United States, more than 98% of all

Division of Gastroenterology, Department of Medicine, Mount Sinai School of Medicine, New York, NY 10029, USA
* Corresponding author. 311 East 79th Street, New York, NY 10075.
E-mail address: lawrence.cohen@nyga.md

Clin Liver Dis 14 (2010) 185–194
doi:10.1016/j.cld.2010.03.003

endoscopies are performed under some form of sedation. In a recent nationwide survey, approximately 65% of the respondents indicated that their standard method of sedation was a benzodiazepine, alone or combined with an opioid.[2] Midazolam was the favored benzodiazepine over diazepam by a wide margin, whereas clinicians used the opioid analgesics meperidine and fentanyl in approximately equal proportions. The remaining endoscopists, approximately 35%, indicated that propofol was their preferred form of sedation. This section reviews the pharmacology of sedation and analgesic drugs commonly used for endoscopic sedation and the pharmacokinetic and pharmacodynamic changes that result from chronic liver disease.

Benzodiazepine

The benzodiazepines, including diazepam and midazolam, are sedative hypnotics that act by selectively attaching to the postsynaptic alpha subunit to enhance channel-gating function of γ-aminobutric acid (GABA). The onset of action for midazolam is between 1 and 2 minutes, the peak effect occurs in 3 to 5 minutes, and its duration of action is 1 to 3 hours. Benzodiazepines have central nervous system effects, including amnesia, hypnosis, muscle-relaxant, and sedative effects. The benzodiazepines are eliminated almost exclusively by the liver. The main determinants of midazolam elimination are the drug metabolizing system (cytochrome P450 enzymes) and the hepatic blood flow. In patients with cirrhosis, decreased protein binding, reduced clearance and metabolism, and increased volume of distribution contribute to a markedly prolonged duration drug half-life.[3,4]

The alterations in pharmacokinetics associated with the use of midazolam in cirrhotic patients have been studied by several investigators. Trouvin and colleagues[5] reported that the disposition of midazolam was nearly unchanged in patients with a moderate degree of liver dysfunction. By comparison, MacGilchrist and colleagues[6] observed a 2-fold prolongation of the elimination half-life of midazolam (3.9 vs 1.6 hours) as a result of decreased clearance in patients with end-stage liver disease. Clinically, recovery time in patients with cirrhosis was prolonged up to 6 hours after administration of midazolam. Chalasani and colleagues[7] compared systemic clearance of midazolam in patients with cirrhosis and portosystemic shunting (created via a transcutaneous intrahepatic portosystemic shunt procedure) with clearance in cirrhotic controls and healthy volunteers. Drug clearance and hepatic extraction of midazolam were reduced 2- to 3-fold, and drug half-life was increased 2.4-fold in the cirrhotic patients with portosystemic shunting compared with the 2 control groups. This study corroborated other reports, indicating that dosing of midazolam should be significantly modified in cirrhotic patients who manifest evidence of significant portosystemic shunting.[7]

In summary, despite significant hepatic metabolism of the benzodiazepines, studies suggest that the pharmacokinetic profile of benzodiazepines administered in single doses has a minimal impact in patients with compensated cirrhosis. In the presence of more severe hepatic dysfunction or significant portosystemic shunting, however, the clinical effects and duration of action of benzodiazepines are more pronounced. It is recommended that benzodiazepines be administered cautiously to patients with decompensated liver disease, especially when administering repeated dosages or prolonged intravenous infusions.

Flumazenil

Flumazenil, due to its high affinity for the benzodiazepine receptor and lack of intrinsic agonist activity, competitively antagonizes the activity of benzodiazepines. Its onset of action and time to peak effect are 2 to 3 minutes and 5 to 8 minutes, respectively.

Flumazenil has a brief duration of action because of rapid redistribution and high liver extraction.[8] The dose of flumazenil needed to reverse the effects of hypnosis and sedation are proportionately less than the dose required to antagonize anxiolysis.

The administration of flumazenil to patients with hepatic encephalopathy has been reported to produce short-term improvement in patients with cirrhosis and hepatic encephalopathy. It is uncertain how long this effect lasts, and there is no evidence that flumazenil has any significant effect on recovery or survival from hepatic encephalopathy.[9]

Opioids

The opioids are frequently used in combination with a benzodiazepine for moderate sedation. Opioids bind to receptors in the central nervous system and act by increasing pain threshold and altering pain perception. The onset of action for meperidine is 5 minutes with the peak effect at 10 minutes and duration of action lasting 2 to 4 hours. The adverse effects of meperidine include hypoventilation, hypotension, lowering of seizure threshold, respiratory depression, decreased tidal volume, nausea, and vomiting. Fentanyl has a somewhat shorter onset of duration (<1 minute) and peak effect (5–8 minutes). The duration of action for fentanyl is 30 to 60 minutes. Adverse effects include hypoventilation, respiratory depression, and decrease in tidal volume (due to chest wall rigidity).[10]

The hepatic clearance of meperidine is prolonged in patients with advanced liver disease. Normeperidine, the major metabolite of meperidine, is also cleared more slowly. With repeated doses of meperidine, toxic levels of normeperidine may accumulate and, especially in patients with renal disease, may result in seizures.[11]

In contrast with meperidine, fentanyl is highly lipid-soluble opioid with a shorter duration of effect due to redistribution into storage sites. It is almost completely metabolized by the liver and as such, its elimination half-life is expected to be prolonged in patients with hepatic dysfunction. Contrary to expectation, however, the available data indicate that fentanyl elimination is not appreciably prolonged in patients with cirrhosis.[11]

Naloxone

Structurally related to morphine, naloxone hydrochloride antagonizes all of the central nervous system effects of the opioids, including ventilatory depression. Naloxone possesses no intrinsic agonist activity. Its onset of action is 1 to 2 minutes and its half-life 30 to 45 minutes. Naloxone is metabolized in the liver by glucuronidation. Patients should receive an initial dose of 0.2 to 0.4 mg (0.5 to 1.0 μg/kg) intravenously every 2 to 3 minutes until the desired response is attained. Supplemental doses may be necessary after 20 to 30 minutes. Careful titration of the dose is required in all patients receiving naloxone and dose modification is not required in patients with chronic liver disease.

Propofol

Propofol (2,6-diisopropyl phenol) is a short-acting sedative that is frequently used for sedation during endoscopic procedures. Propofol acts on the GABAergic neurons in the brain, resulting in sedation and anesthesia with little or no analgesic effect. Its onset of action coincides with 1 arm-brain circulation, approximately 30 to 45 seconds, whereas its duration of effect is 4 to 8 minutes. The adverse effects of propofol include hypotension, tachycardia, hypoventilation, and prolonged QT interval. The properties that make propofol an attractive sedative are its quick onset of action, rapid clearance after dosing for endoscopic procedures, and faster recovery. Propofol has synergistic effects with benzodiazepines and narcotics, and extra caution should be exercised when administering an opioid or benzodiazepine to a patient who has recently received propofol.

Propofol is rapidly metabolized in the liver by conjugation to glucuronide and sulfate, resulting in water-soluble compounds that are then readily excreted by the kidney. Extrahepatic metabolism of propofol has been demonstrated, with up to a 30% reduction in propofol concentration resulting from first pass clearance through the lungs. Its pharmacokinetic profile is affected by weight, gender, age, and concomitant disease. The presence of chronic liver disease, however, has been reported not to significantly alter propofol's pharmacokinetic profile.[12]

HEPATIC ENCEPHALOPATHY AND ENDOSCOPIC SEDATION

Hepatic encephalopathy refers to a complex neuropsychiatric syndrome that may complicate acute or chronic liver disease. It is defined by changes in mental status that range from subtle alterations in intellectual function and minimal personality changes to altered level of consciousness (including coma), neuromuscular disorders, and seizure. A subclinical stage of hepatic encephalopathy, termed, *minimal hepatic encephalopathy (MHE)*, has been described that is unrecognizable during routine examination but is distinguishable by neuropsychiatric testing. Some investigators estimate that this condition affects up to 60% of individuals with cirrhosis.[1] MHE is significant for 2 reasons. First, it predisposes to the clinically overt form of encephalopathy. Patients with MHE have a 3- to 4-fold increased risk of developing overt hepatic encephalopathy compared with cirrhotics without MHE. Second, it may have an impact on daily activities, such as driving ability, tasks requiring fine motor skills, and the performance of work-related activities.[13,14]

Establishing the diagnosis of MHE can be difficult because a diagnostic gold standard is not currently available. Several psychometric tests, including the number connection, block design, and digit symbol tests, have been used to identify MHE.[15] These tests assess various areas of cognition as well as mental and motor speed. The diagnosis of MHE is based on the results of neuropsychological testing and the exclusion of other metabolic and neurologic abnormalities.

The cause of hepatic encephalopathy is believed to be multifactorial. Activation of the GABA receptors in the brain seems to contribute to encephalopathy, helping to explain why the GABA receptor antagonist, flumanzenil, produces short-term improvement in the symptoms of encephalopathy. Known precipitants of hepatic encephalopathy include gastrointestinal bleeding, hypovolemia, infection, and drugs used to produce sedation or analgesia. The desire to avoid drugs that could potentially worsen encephalopathy has focused attention on the method of sedation used for patients with chronic liver disease.

The effect of sedation drugs on hepatic encephalopathy has been examined in several studies. Assy and colleagues[16] evaluated the effect of midazolam on neuropsychiatric function in cirrhotic patients and healthy controls undergoing EGD. Nine of 10 cirrhotic patients had an abnormal baseline number connection test, and all 10 had an abnormal test 2 hours post treatment. In contrast, none of the healthy control subjects had an abnormal number connection test result at baseline or after recovery from sedation.

Vasudevan and colleagues[17] administered midazolam (5 mg intravenously) to cirrhotic and healthy controls, recording number connection test results at baseline and 2 hours post sedation. The baseline and postsedation scores for cirrhotic patients were 43 and 60 seconds, respectively, compared with 34 and 33 seconds in the control group. The proportion of patients with a postsedation prolonged score was significantly greater among the cirrhotic patients than the controls. The results of these 2 trials suggest that cirrhotic patients are more sensitive to the sedative effect of benzodiazepines and that clinicians should be attentive to the development or worsening of encephalopathy in cirrhotic patients who receive a benzodiazepine for endoscopic sedation.

In another study, Amoros and colleagues[18] compared the effect of propofol in compensated cirrhotic patients without overt evidence of encephalopathy and in healthy controls. The psychometric hepatic encephalopathy score, a battery of 4 psychometric tests, along with the critical flicker frequency (CFF), were used to diagnose MHE. All patients underwent EGD with nurse-administered propofol titrated to deep sedation. Thirteen of 20 cirrhotic patients had evidence of MHE before endoscopy. Post procedure, no differences in CFF were observed among the cirrhotic patients, suggesting that deep sedation with propofol does not provoke overt hepatic encephalopathy, even among those with evidence of MHE at baseline.

GENERAL PRINCIPLES OF SEDATION

Continuum of Sedation

Sedation may be defined a drug-induced alteration in the level of consciousness. This altered state of consciousness occurs along a continuum that ranges from anxiolysis to unconsciousness. Four stages of sedation have been described: minimal, moderate, deep, and general anesthesia.[19] These levels of sedation are defined based on a stimulus/response relationship. For example, minimal sedation or anxiolysis is defined by a normal response to spoken commands. At the other end of the continuum, general anesthesia is defined by the total absence of response, even to painful stimuli. Moderate sedation (responsiveness to verbal or light tactile stimulus) and deep sedation (responsiveness to deep painful stimulus) represent levels that are in-between these 2 extremes. With increasing depth of sedation, there is greater potential for some compromise of cardiovascular function, ventilatory drive, and an ability to maintain an intact airway. Moderate sedation is generally associated with preservation of cardiorespiratory function and an intact airway. As such, it is generally considered an acceptable target level of sedation by nonanesthesiologists.

Sedation is a dynamic process, subject to fluctuations up and down during a single examination. For example, the administration of a noxious stimulus during an endoscopic procedure may cause a sedated patient to awaken. Due to the potential for oversedation, clinicians should be able to rescue patients who become more deeply sedated than intended. In practical terms, this means that a physician targeting moderate sedation should possess the skills to resuscitate a patient in deep sedation, and likewise, one that is targeting deep sedation should be able to rescue a patient from general anesthesia. The practical implications of this principle are beyond the scope of this review and interested readers are directed to more comprehensive reviews of the subject.[20]

Preprocedure Assessment

Prior to the initiation of endoscopy, a preprocedure assessment should always be performed. The goal of this evaluation is the identification of elements of the patient's history or physical examination that could have an impact on sedation. Factors in the history that should be considered include cardiac or pulmonary disease; neurologic disease or seizures; obstructive airway disease or sleep apnea; prior unfavorable reaction to anesthesia or sedation; current medications; history of allergy to drugs, food, or latex; and a history of alcohol or drug abuse. Patients with known or suspected chronic liver disease should also be queried concerning a history of bleeding esophageal varices, easy bruising, ascites, and hepatic encephalopathy. The examination should include the patient's vital signs, weight, cardiopulmonary auscultation, level of consciousness, and airway assessment. Certain anatomic features of the airway, including obesity, short thick neck, cervical spine disease, decreased hyoid-mental distance, and structural abnormalities of the oropharynx, are associated with a more difficult tracheal intubation. The Mallampati score, based on an ability to visualize the faucial pillar and base of the tongue on maximal mouth opening, is also a useful tool for predicting a difficult intubation. Evidence of hepatic encephalopathy and the presence of ascites or peripheral edema should be ascertained.

Another important component of the preprocedure evaluation is assessment of a patient's American Society for Anesthesiologists (ASA) physical status classification. The ASA classification categorizes patients into 1 of 5 categories and has been shown to predict a patient's risk of sedation.[21] Normal healthy patients without organic, physiologic, or psychiatric disease are considered ASA I. In general, patients classified as ASA I and II are considered appropriate for sedation and monitoring by a gastroenterologist. There is a lack of agreement concerning the management of ASA III patients; the decision over whether or not a specific patient is suitable for sedation by an endoscopist is best left to a clinician.[20] It is recommended that an anesthesia consultation be obtained before performing endoscopy on patients who are classified as ASA IV or V. Furthermore, the guidelines also recommend consultation with an anesthesiologist in certain situations, such as for patients with alcohol or substance abuse, in emergency cases, or for patients who experienced prior difficulties with anesthesia or conscious sedation. Most patients with chronic liver disease and hepatic dysfunction are ASA III, although those with overt signs of hepatic encephalopathy are ASA IV. Fasting before endoscopy is important to allow an unimpeded view of the gastric mucosa as well as to prevent pulmonary aspiration during sedation. There are many recommendations on what constitutes an adequate period of fasting before sedation, because no trial has demonstrated a relationship between the length of fast and aspiration.[20,22] The ASA guidelines recommend a 2-hour fast if a patient is drinking clear liquids and a 6-hour fast if a patient had a light meal.

In healthy individuals, laboratory testing is not routinely required before endoscopy. In patients with chronic liver disease and a history of bleeding, a baseline hemoglobin, platelet count, and prothrombin time International normalized ratio (INR) may be advisable before endoscopy in the event that tissue sampling or polypectomy is required or a patient requires urgent tracheal intubation.

Monitoring

Monitoring devices should be checked to confirm that they are functioning properly before the initiation of sedation. Appropriate equipment for standard sedation includes the use of pulse oximetry, automated noninvasive blood pressure, and electrographic monitors. Monitoring of patients should begin before the commencement of sedation and be maintained throughout the procedure and recovery until patients are cleared for discharge. Effective monitoring should also include visual assessment of patients in addition to measurement of physiologic parameters. Appropriate intervention should be instituted at the earliest indication of physiologic instability to avoid a more significant adverse event. For example, hypoxemia should be addressed promptly by assessing patient ventilatory status, providing airway intervention using chin lift or jaw thrust, and, when necessary, increasing the concentration of inspired oxygen.

In addition to equipment, appropriate monitoring requires that a nurse or assistant be present throughout the procedure. This individual should be trained and capable of interpreting physiologic parameters, understand the stages of sedation, possess the ability to intervene in the event of a complication, and be certified in basic or advanced cardiac life support. During procedures that are performed under moderate sedation, an assistant or nurse may perform brief interruptible tasks as necessary. When deep sedation is the target, however, this individual must be dedicated exclusively to monitoring the patient and may not have other responsibilities. At least 1 individual involved in the procedure should be certified in advanced cardiac life support and be capable of establishing an airway for positive-pressure ventilation.

Level of sedation should be assessed periodically throughout every procedure. Several sedation scales have been developed for this purpose, including the Ramsay Sedation Scale[23] and the Modified Observer's Assessment of Alertness and Sedation Scale (MOAAS).[24] The MOAAS scale classifies sedation on a 6-point scale (0 through 5), with 5 representing a patient who is fully awake and 2, 3, and 4 reflecting moderate sedation, 1 deep sedation, and 0 general anesthesia. The MOAAS score should be recorded before the start of the procedure and periodically throughout the procedure and recovery until the patient is ready for discharge.

Emergency equipment should be readily available wherever sedation is administered. Necessary items include oral and nasal airways, mask and Ambu bag, and a defibrillator. When deep sedation is targeted, advanced airway equipment, including laryngoscopes, endotracheal tubes, and laryngeal mask airways, should also be available. A list of emergency medications appropriate for emergency use has been summarized elsewhere.[20]

The use of supplemental oxygen is routinely recommended by the ASA[19] and American Society for Gastrointestinal Endoscopy.[25] There are no data, however, to show that use of supplemental oxygen reduces cardiopulmonary complications. Furthermore, supplemental oxygen may actually delay recognition of hypoventilation. Supplemental oxygen should be readily available whenever endoscopic sedation is administered.

Recovery and Discharge

After the completion of endoscopy, patients should continue to be monitored until they are ready for discharge. The individual assigned responsibility for monitoring during recovery should assess a patient's level of consciousness, heart rate, blood pressure, and oxygenation as well presence of pain or discomfort. These parameters should be recorded until they have returned to the preprocedure level. Patients receiving naloxone or flumazenil should be monitored for as long as 2 hours to avoid the risk of a complication due to resedation.

Suitability for discharge should be assessed using standardized criteria. One of the more commonly used discharge scales is the Aldrete scoring system. The Aldrete encompasses 5 parameters: respiration, oxygen saturation, blood pressure, consciousness, and activity. A patient suitable for discharge should be able to dress and walk independently. Prior to leaving the endoscopy facility, patients should receive written instructions with regard to diet, activity, medication changes, and plan for follow-up. Further, patients should be provided with information on how to reach a person 24 hours a day should a complication arise. Patients should also be escorted home by a responsible individual.

SPECIAL CONSIDERATIONS

Unsedated Endoscopy

An alternative approach to upper endoscopy in high-risk patients is to perform an unsedated examination. Darwin and colleagues[26] prospectively evaluated the

17. Vasudevan AE, Goh KL, Bulgiba AM. Impairment of psychomotor responses after conscious sedation in cirrhotic patients undergoing therapeutic upper GI endoscopy. Am J Gastroenterol 2002;97:1717–21.
18. Amoros A, Aparicio JR, Garmendia M, et al. Deep sedation with propofol does not precipitate hepatic. Gastrointest Endosc 2009;70(2):262–8.
19. Gross JB, Bailey PL, Connis RT, et al. Practice guidelines for sedation and analgesia by non-anesthesiologists. Anesthesiology 2002;96(4):1004–17.
20. Cohen LB, DeLegge M, Kochman M, et al. AGA Institute review on endoscopic sedation. Gastroenterology 2007;133:675–701.
21. Dripps RD, Lamont A, Eckenhoff JE. The role of anesthesia in surgical mortality. JAMA 1961;178:261–6.
22. Warner MA, Caplan RA, Epstein BS, et al. Practice guidelines for preoperative fasting and the use of pharmacologic agents to reduce the risk of pulmonary aspiration: application to healthy patients undergoing elective procedures: a report by the American Society of Anesthesiologist Task Force on Preoperative Fasting. Anesthesiology 1999;90:896–905.
23. Ramsay M, Savege T, Simpson B. Controlled sedation with alphaxalone-alphadolone. BMJ 1974;2(5920):656–9.
24. Chernik DA, Gillings D, Laine H, et al. Validity and reliability of the Observer's Assessment of Alertness/Sedation Scale: study with intravenous midazolam. J Clin Psychopharmacol 1990;10(4):244–51.
25. Waring JP, Baron TH, Hirota WK, et al. Guidelines for conscious sedation and monitoring during gastrointestinal endoscopy. Gastrointest Endosc 2003;58(3): 317–22.
26. Darwin P, Zangara J, Heller T, et al. Unsedated esophagoscopy for the diagnosis of esophageal varices in patients with cirrhosis. Endoscopy 2000;32:971–3.
27. Evans LT, Saberi S, Kim HM, et al. Pharyngeal anesthesia during sedated EGDs: is "the spray" beneficial? A meta-analysis and systematic review. Gastrointest Endosc 2006;63(6):761–6.
28. Abraham NS, Fallone CA, Mayrand S, et al. Sedation versus no sedation in the performance of diagnostic upper gastrointestinal endoscopy: a Canadian randomized controlled cost-outcome study. Am J Gastroenterol 2004;99(9): 1692–9.
29. Weston BR, Chadalawada V, Chalasani N, et al. Nurse-administered propofol versus midazolam and meperidine for upper endoscopy in cirrhotic patients. Am J Gastroenterol 2003;98(11):2440–7.

Current Staging and Diagnosis of Gastroesophageal Varices

Nayantara Coelho-Prabhu, MD, Patrick S. Kamath, MD*

KEYWORDS

• Esophageal varices • Gastric varices • Diagnosis • Staging

Portal hypertension is defined as an increase in hepatic sinusoidal pressure to 6 mm Hg or higher. Cirrhosis is the most common cause of portal hypertension in the western world and results from increased resistance to blood flow at the hepatic sinusoidal level.

ANATOMY AND PATHOPHYSIOLOGY

The portal venous system provides venous drainage for the entire gastrointestinal tract except for the proximal esophagus and very distal rectum, but does drain the spleen, pancreas, and gallbladder. The splenic vein and superior mesenteric vein coalesce to form the portal vein behind the neck of the pancreas. The inferior mesenteric vein drains into the splenic vein and the left gastric vein usually drains into the origin of the portal vein. The portal vein then runs in the gastrohepatic ligament to the hilum of the liver where it divides into right and left portal veins, which then further branch out into portal venules feeding into hepatic sinusoids. The sinusoids drain distally into the right, middle, and left hepatic veins, which empty into the retrohepatic inferior vena cava.

Portal hypertension results from a combination of increased resistance to blood flow in the liver and an increase in the portal blood flow. When cirrhosis develops, the resistance through the normally compliant hepatic circulatory bed increases, which leads to portal hypertension. Nodular regeneration and fibrosis as a result of inflammation and scarring lead to structural changes, which are largely irreversible. An excess of vasoconstrictor substances, such as endothelin-1, and a reduction in vasodilators,

This work was not supported by any grants.
The authors have no financial disclosures or conflicts.
Division of Gastroenterology and Hepatology, Mayo Clinic Rochester, 200 First Street SW, Rochester, MN 55905, USA
* Corresponding author.
E-mail address: kamath.patrick@mayo.edu

Clin Liver Dis 14 (2010) 195–208
doi:10.1016/j.cld.2010.03.006

such as nitric oxide (NO), are also contributory factors. Also, the hepatic stellate cells, which lie in the perisinusoidal space of Disse and are usually quiescent, are activated and contract the sinusoids thereby increasing intrahepatic resistance.

In contrast, there is an increase in NO production in the splanchnic vascular bed leading to vasodilation and increased blood flow.[1] The systemic vascular dilation leads to development of a hyperdynamic circulatory system in patients with cirrhosis. Increased splanchnic flow causes increased flow into the portal veins, thereby increasing the portal pressures and worsening the portal hypertension.

Collaterals usually exist between the portal venous system and the systemic veins. However, the resistance in the portal bed is lower than in the collateral circulation and so blood flows from the systemic bed into the portal bed. However, when portal hypertension develops, the portal pressure is higher than systemic venous pressure, and this leads to reversal of flow in these collaterals. Eventually, there is angiogenesis and development of new collaterals and increase in the size of the collaterals in an attempt to decompress the portal circulation. **Table 1** shows the locations and vessels involved in the collaterals. Unfortunately these collaterals are insufficient to decompress the hypertension. The collaterals lead to complications of portal hypertension including variceal hemorrhage and encephalopathy.

Esophageal varices form when the hepatic vein pressure gradient (HVPG) is greater than or equal to 10 mm Hg. The gastroesophageal (GE) area is the main site of formation of varices (**Fig. 1**).[2] The gastric portions of the varices extend down from the GE junction for 2 to 3 cm into the fundus. Along the lesser curvature, they drain into the left gastric or coronary vein and into the portal vein. Along the greater curvature, they drain through the short gastric veins into the splenic vein. Dilation of these veins results in gastric varices. In the lower 2 to 3 cm of the esophagus, the collaterals in the submucosa do not communicate with the periesophageal veins and cannot easily be decompressed. Above this level, for another 3 to 4 cm, the esophageal varices are connected to the periesophageal veins via perforating veins and thus are able to decompress into them and into the azygous vein. Above this, esophageal varices can extend upwards for another 10 cm, but easily decompress through the perforating veins, which is the reason that esophageal varices bleed only at the lower end of the esophagus and therefore therapy should also be targeted to this site.

All patients diagnosed with cirrhosis of the liver should be screened for esophageal varices. Varices should be suspected in all patients with spider nevi, jaundice, palmar erythema, Dupuytren's contractures, testicular atrophy, loss of secondary sexual characteristics, splenomegaly, ascites, encephalopathy, and caput medusae.

DIAGNOSIS OF GASTROESOPHAGEAL VARICES

Varices can be detected using various techniques.

Table 1
Location and blood vessels of collaterals between the portal and systemic venous systems

Location	Portal System	Systemic System
Distal esophagus and proximal stomach	Short gastric and left gastric (coronary) vein	Azygous vein
Rectum	Inferior mesenteric vein	Pudendal vein
Umbilicus (caput medusae)	Left portal vein	Umbilical vein
Retroperitoneum	Mesenteric veins	Renal vein or iliac veins

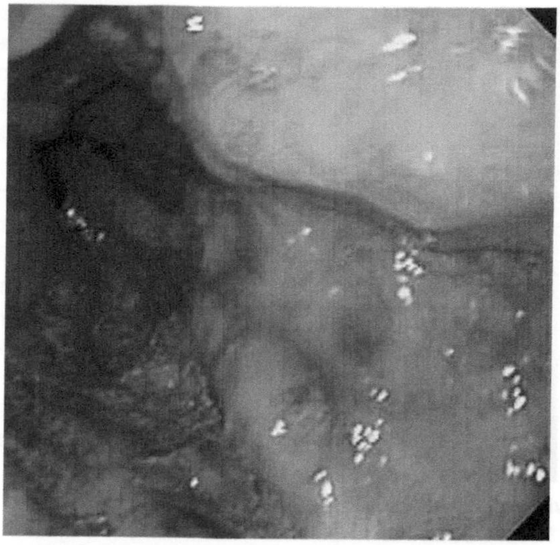

Fig. 1. Endoscopic image showing esophageal varices at the gastroesophageal junction.

Esophagogastroduodenoscopy

Esophagogastroduodenoscopy (EGD) is the most common method to diagnose varices. All patients with a diagnosis of cirrhosis should be screened for varices with an EGD. If no varices are seen, repeat EGD should be performed in 2 to 3 years. If small varices are seen, repeat EGD should be performed in 1 to 2 years or earlier if patients show evidence of decompensation.[3]

An EGD is considered the gold standard for diagnosis of GE varices because it enables the endoscopist to obtain a direct view of the varices and decide on the management by assessing the size of the varices and the presence of red wale marks and cherry spots. Also, if prophylactic or therapeutic variceal banding is warranted, it can be performed at the same sitting.

Examination for varices must be performed during withdrawal of the endoscope.[4] The esophagus must be maximally inflated with air after the stomach is completely aspirated, which flattens out any esophageal folds that may masquerade as varices. Varices must be described as to their location in the esophagus (lower, middle, or upper) and their size (small [<5 mm, **Fig. 2**] or large [>5 mm, **Fig. 3**]). For reasons alluded to earlier, only varices in the lower esophagus are at risk for bleeding, and therefore should be graded and described. Grading of varices are described later in this article.

Ultrathin endoscopy can be performed without sedation and is an option for patients in whom sedation is contraindicated. There have been small studies thus far comparing the efficacy of this scope to a regular EGD scope. Darwin and colleagues[5] found varices in 9 of 15 subjects with cirrhosis but there was no EGD performed simultaneously to confirm this. Madhotra and colleagues[6] studied 28 subjects who had both types of endoscopy and found ultrathin endoscopy had a sensitivity and negative predictive value of 100% with a specificity and positive predictive value of 93% for the detection of esophageal varices. The procedure was also well tolerated. Further studies are needed before this becomes the standard of practice.

Capsule Endoscopy

Capsule endoscopy (CE) uses the PillCam Eso (Given Imaging Ltd, Yoqneam, Israel), which measures 26 by 11 mm. Initial pilot studies demonstrated the safety,

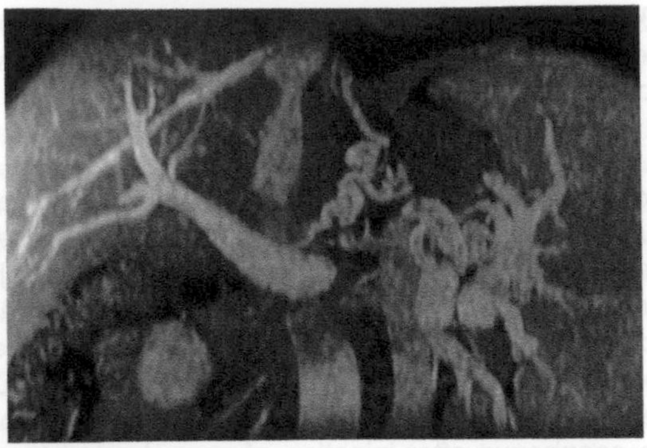

Fig. 7. MRI image showing the portal venous system and esophageal varices.

was higher in subjects with portal hypertension than normal controls[42] and highest at midnight, a fact that helps guide the timing of beta blocker treatment.[43]

Matsuo and colleagues[44] evaluated the use of gadolinium-enhanced MRI to detect and grade esophageal varices. Seventy-two subjects underwent MRI and EGD (reference). The sensitivity of gadolinium-enhanced MRI to detect varices was 81%. A significant correlation was also found in the grading of varices between the MRI and endoscopic images. MRI with a transesophageal probe has also been studied[45] and found to be feasible, but further patient satisfaction and cost-effectiveness studies are needed. Willmann and colleagues[46] found MR angiography was equivalent to EUS for detection of gastric fundal varices.

GRADING OF GASTROESOPHAGEAL VARICES

Esophageal Varices

Endoscopic grading of esophageal varices is quite subjective and interobserver variability exists.[47–49] Three grading systems exist: by Dagradi[50] (1972); by the Japanese Research Society for Portal Hypertension (JRSPH, 1980)[51]; and by the North Italian Endoscopy Club for the Study and Treatment of Esophageal varices (NIEC, 1988).[52]

Dagradi classified esophageal varices into five grades:

I: 1 to 2 mm in diameter, and straight or sigmoid shaped
II: Similar to I but visible without occluding blood flow in the vessel
III: 3 to 4 mm in diameter and straight or tortuous
IV: 4 to 5 mm in diameter, tortuous, often coiled, seen in all quadrants of esophagus
V: Greater than 5 mm in diameter, tightly packed, grape-like, covered by thin, wrinkled mucosa, with overlying cherry red spots and telangiectasias.

The JRSPH system grades varices based on location, form color, and red color sign:

- The location of varices may be upper, middle, or lower third of the esophagus or upper stomach.
- The form of the varices is classified as small and straight (F1), enlarged and tortuous (F2), or large and coil shaped (F3).
- The color of the varices is graded as white (Cw) or blue (Cb).
- Also included is the presence of the red color sign (RC) that are dilated, small vessels (red wale sign), and telangiectasias or cherry-red spots on the surface of the varices (**Fig. 8**).

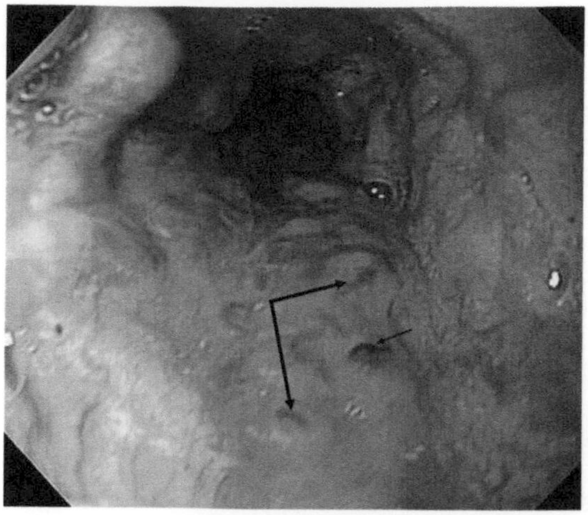

Fig. 8. Endoscopic image showing large varices with cherry red spot (*thin arrow*) and red wale markings (*thick arrows*).

The NIEC index takes into account the following

- The Child-Pugh class of cirrhosis (A, B, or C)
- Variceal size (small, medium, or large)
- Presence of red color signs (absent, mild, moderate, or severe).

Of these variables, variceal size and red color signs are the most important.[53] Rigo and colleagues[54] prospectively followed 320 subjects with varices and classified each subject according to each of these systems. They found that the JRSPH and NIEC classifications were highly specific to predict variceal bleeding (93.4% and 94.8%, respectively) but not sensitive. All three systems had low positive predictive values. The investigators concluded that although these classifications can identify patients with high risk for bleeding, few patients that will bleed fall into these high-risk groups. Nevertheless, the NIEC and JRSPH classifications are commonly used to describe varices in investigative and clinical settings.

The Baveno I consensus conference[55] in 1992 recommended that esophageal varices be classified as small (<5 mm) and large (>5 mm). Roughly, 5 mm is the size of an open biopsy forceps. Cales and colleagues[56] confirmed this cutoff as being optimal to differentiate small from large varices. The guidelines for primary prophylaxis differ based on whether varices are graded as small or large.[3] Patients with large-size varices, Child-Pugh class C cirrhosis, and red color signs on the varices have the highest risk for bleeding within 1 year.[52,53]

Gastric Varices

Gastric varices are classified by Sarin[57] as follows

- GOV1: Type 1 GE varices (extend 2–5 cm below the GE junction and in continuity with esophageal varices)
- GOV2: Type 2 GE varices (in the fundus of the stomach and in continuity with esophageal varices)
- IGV1: Type 1 isolated gastric varices (isolated gastric varices in the fundus of the stomach in the absence of esophageal varices)
- IGV2: Type 2 isolated gastric varices (in the gastric body, antrum or pylorus).

20. Kassem AM, Salama ZA, Zakaria MS, et al. Endoscopic ultrasonographic study of the azygous vein before and after endoscopic obliteration of esophagogastric varices by injection sclerotherapy. Endoscopy 2000;32:630.
21. Miller L, Banson FL, Bazir K, et al. Risk of esophageal variceal bleeding based on endoscopic ultrasound evaluation of the sum of esophageal variceal cross-sectional surface area. Am J Gastroenterol 2003;98:454.
22. Konishi Y, Nakamura T, Kida H, et al. Catheter US probe EUS evaluation of gastric cardia and perigastric vascular structures to predict esophageal variceal recurrence. Gastrointest Endosc 2002;55:197.
23. Ito K, Matsutani S, Maruyama H, et al. Study of hemodynamic changes in portal systemic shunts and their relation to variceal relapse after endoscopic variceal ligation combined with ethanol sclerotherapy. J Gastroenterol 2006;41:119.
24. Kuramochi A, Imazu H, Kakutani H, et al. Color Doppler endoscopic ultrasonography in identifying groups at a high-risk of recurrence of esophageal varices after endoscopic treatment. J Gastroenterol 2007;42:219.
25. Escorsell A, Bordas JM, Feu F, et al. Endoscopic assessment of variceal volume and wall tension in cirrhotic patients: effects of pharmacological therapy. Gastroenterology 1997;113:1640.
26. Pontes JM, Leitao MC, Portela F, et al. Endosonographic Doppler-guided manometry of esophageal varices: experimental validation and clinical feasibility. Endoscopy 2002;34:966.
27. de Paulo GA, Ardengh JC, Nakao FS, et al. Treatment of esophageal varices: a randomized controlled trial comparing endoscopic sclerotherapy and EUS-guided sclerotherapy of esophageal collateral veins. Gastrointest Endosc 2006;63:396.
28. Romero-Castro R, Pellicer-Bautista FJ, Jimenez-Saenz M, et al. EUS-guided injection of cyanoacrylate in perforating feeding veins in gastric varices: results in 5 cases. Gastrointest Endosc 2007;66:402.
29. Cottone M, D'Amico G, Maringhini A, et al. Predictive value of ultrasonography in the screening of non-ascitic cirrhotic patients with large varices. J Ultrasound Med 1986;5:189.
30. Schepis F, Camma C, Niceforo D, et al. Which patients with cirrhosis should undergo endoscopic screening for esophageal varices detection? Hepatology 2001;33:333.
31. Van Gansbeke D, Avni EF, Delcour C, et al. Sonographic features of portal vein thrombosis. AJR Am J Roentgenol 1985;144:749.
32. Kazemi F, Kettaneh A, N'Kontchou G, et al. Liver stiffness measurement selects patients with cirrhosis at risk of bearing large oesophageal varices. J Hepatol 2006;45:230.
33. Vizzutti F, Arena U, Romanelli RG, et al. Liver stiffness measurement predicts severe portal hypertension in patients with HCV-related cirrhosis. Hepatology 2007;45:1290.
34. Foucher J, Chanteloup E, Vergniol J, et al. Diagnosis of cirrhosis by transient elastography (FibroScan): a prospective study. Gut 2006;55:403.
35. Castera L, Le Bail B, Roudot-Thoraval F, et al. Early detection in routine clinical practice of cirrhosis and oesophageal varices in chronic hepatitis C: comparison of transient elastography (FibroScan) with standard laboratory tests and non-invasive scores. J Hepatol 2009;50:59.
36. Kim YJ, Raman SS, Yu NC, et al. Esophageal varices in cirrhotic patients: evaluation with liver CT. AJR Am J Roentgenol 2007;188:139.

37. Kim SH, Kim YJ, Lee JM, et al. Esophageal varices in patients with cirrhosis: multidetector CT esophagography–comparison with endoscopy. Radiology 2007;242:759.
38. Perri RE, Chiorean MV, Fidler JL, et al. A prospective evaluation of computerized tomographic (CT) scanning as a screening modality for esophageal varices. Hepatology 2008;47:1587.
39. Willmann JK, Weishaupt D, Bohm T, et al. Detection of submucosal gastric fundal varices with multi-detector row CT angiography. Gut 2003;52:886.
40. Finn JP, Kane RA, Edelman RR, et al. Imaging of the portal venous system in patients with cirrhosis: MR angiography vs duplex Doppler sonography. AJR Am J Roentgenol 1993;161:989.
41. Wu MT, Pan HB, Chen C, et al. Azygos blood flow in cirrhosis: measurement with MR imaging and correlation with variceal hemorrhage. Radiology 1996;198:457.
42. Sugano S, Yamamoto K, Takamura N, et al. Azygos venous blood flow while fasting, postprandially, and after endoscopic variceal ligation, measured by magnetic resonance imaging. J Gastroenterol 1999;34:310.
43. Sugano S, Yamamoto K, Sasao K, et al. Daily variation of azygos and portal blood flow and the effect of propranolol administration once an evening in cirrhotics. J Hepatol 2001;34:26.
44. Matsuo M, Kanematsu M, Kim T, et al. Esophageal varices: diagnosis with gadolinium-enhanced MR imaging of the liver for patients with chronic liver damage. AJR Am J Roentgenol 2003;180:461.
45. Annet L, Peeters F, Horsmans Y, et al. Esophageal varices: evaluation with transesophageal MR imaging—initial experience. Radiology 2006;238:167.
46. Willmann JK, Bauerfeind P, Boehm T, et al. [Contrast-enhanced MR angiography for differentiation between perigastric and submucosal gastric fundal varices]. Rofo 2003;175:507 [in German].
47. Bendtsen F, Skovgaard LT, Sorensen TI, et al. Agreement among multiple observers on endoscopic diagnosis of esophageal varices before bleeding. Hepatology 1990;11:341.
48. Cales P, Pascal JP. Gastroesophageal endoscopic features in cirrhosis: comparison of intracenter and intercenter observer variability. Gastroenterology 1990;99: 1189.
49. Sauerbruch T, Kleber G. Upper gastrointestinal endoscopy in patients with portal hypertension. Endoscopy 1992;24:45.
50. Dagradi AE. The natural history of esophageal varices in patients with alcoholic liver cirrhosis. An endoscopic and clinical study. Am J Gastroenterol 1972;57: 520.
51. Idezuki Y. General rules for recording endoscopic findings of esophagogastric varices (1991). Japanese Society for Portal Hypertension. World J Surg 1995; 19:420.
52. Brocchi E, Caletti G, Brambilla G, et al. Prediction of the first variceal hemorrhage in patients with cirrhosis of the liver and esophageal varices. A prospective multicenter study. N Engl J Med 1988;319:983.
53. Merkel C, Zoli M, Siringo S, et al. Prognostic indicators of risk for first variceal bleeding in cirrhosis: a multicenter study in 711 patients to validate and improve the North Italian Endoscopic Club (NIEC) index. Am J Gastroenterol 2000;95: 2915.
54. Rigo GP, Merighi A, Chahin NJ, et al. A prospective study of the ability of three endoscopic classifications to predict hemorrhage from esophageal varices. Gastrointest Endosc 1992;38:425.

55. de Franchis R, Pascal JP, Ancona E, et al. Definitions, methodology and therapeutic strategies in portal hypertension. A Consensus Development Workshop, Baveno, Lake Maggiore, Italy, April 5 and 6, 1990. J Hepatol 1992;15:256.
56. Cales P, Oberti F, Bernard-Chabert B, et al. Evaluation of Baveno recommendations for grading esophageal varices. J Hepatol 2003;39:657.
57. Sarin SK, Lahoti D, Saxena SP, et al. Prevalence, classification and natural history of gastric varices: a long-term follow-up study in 568 portal hypertension patients. Hepatology 1992;16:1343.
58. de Franchis R. Updating consensus in portal hypertension: report of the Baveno III Consensus Workshop on definitions, methodology and therapeutic strategies in portal hypertension. J Hepatol 2000;33:846.

Capsule Endoscopy in Portal Hypertension

Emanuele Rondonotti, MD, PhD, Federica Villa, MD,
Alessandra Dell' Era, MD, PhD, Gian Eugenio Tontini, MD,
Roberto de Franchis, MD*

KEYWORDS

- Portal hypertension • Capsule endoscopy
- Esophageal capsule endoscopy • Gastroscopy

The term portal hypertension (PH) was first introduced by Gilbert and Carnot in 1902 to describe a clinical syndrome characterized by ascites, splenomegaly, and esophageal hemorrhage.[1] The mechanism causing these symptoms is the increased blood pressure in the portal system. The portal pressure is normally estimated by measuring the hepatic venous pressure gradient (HVPG). The HVPG is the difference between the wedged hepatic venous pressure (WHVP), which reflects the pressure of hepatic sinusoids, and the free hepatic venous pressure (FHVP). The HVPG normally ranges between 3 and 6 mm Hg.[2] Clinically significant portal hypertension is defined by HVPG greater than 10 mm Hg because the development of ascites, varices, and variceal bleeding usually occurs above this threshold.[3]

The most common cause of portal hypertension is liver cirrhosis. Although the exact prevalence of cirrhosis worldwide is unknown, it was estimated at 0.15% or 400,000 in the United States,[4] accounting for more than 25,000 deaths and 373,000 hospital discharges in 1998.[5] Similar numbers have been reported from Europe, and numbers are even higher in most Asian and African countries where chronic viral hepatitis B or C is frequent. Because compensated cirrhosis often goes undetected for prolonged periods of time, a reasonable estimate is that up to 1% of the world population may have histologic cirrhosis[6] and may develop portal hypertension with time.

CAPSULE ENDOSCOPY IN PORTAL HYPERTENSION: WHY?

Portal hypertension, regardless of its cause, results in blood retention in the portal area and in the formation of a collateral circulation that directly connects the portal vessels to the general circulation, bypassing the liver. The common sites of collateral formation are between the mesenteric and rectal veins, within the abdominal wall around the umbilicus and in the retroperitoneal space. From the clinical and hemodynamic point of view, the

Università degli Studi di Milano, IRCCS Ca' Granda Ospedale Policlinico Foundation, Gastroenterologia 3, Pad Beretta EST, Via F. Sforza 35, Milano 20122, Italy
* Corresponding author.
E-mail address: roberto.defranchis@unimi.it

Clin Liver Dis 14 (2010) 209–220
doi:10.1016/j.cld.2010.03.004

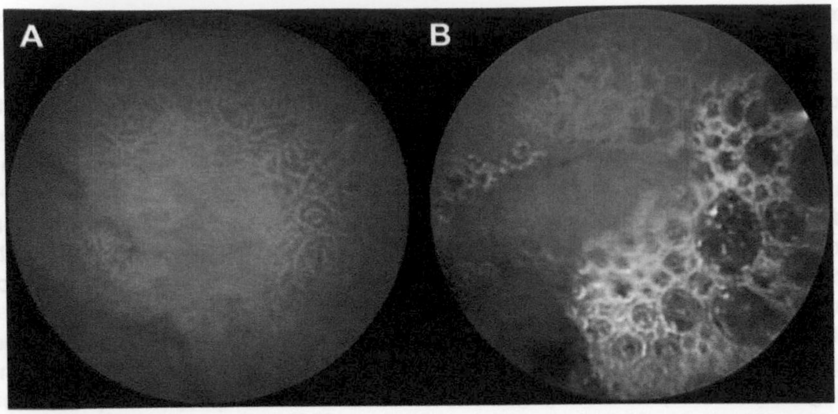

Fig. 2. PHE seen at capsule endoscopy. Edematous mucosa with herring roe appearance (*A*) and hyperemic edematous areas (*B*).

be also used to evaluate the esophagus.[40–42] This technique allows the capsule to be moved up and down the esophagus by gently moving the string, to obtain a clear view of the distal esophagus. In addition, due to its 8 hours battery life, the string capsule can be retrieved via the patient's mouth, and after cleaning and disinfection can be stored and re-used to examine several patients. The string capsule is mostly used to evaluate patients with signs of gastroesophageal reflux disease, dysphagia, or Barrett esophagus.[41,42] To the best of our knowledge, there is only 1 full paper[40] that describes this technique for patients with esophageal varices. Although the performance of the string capsule in recognizing the presence of varices was impressive (96% sensitivity, 100% specificity, positive and negative predictive values 100% and 83%, respectively) in this study, the limited sample size made it difficult to reach any firm conclusion.

Almost all data regarding the usefulness of capsule endoscopy for the assessment of portal hypertension is derived from studies that used PillCam-ESO (Given Imaging Yoqneam, Israel), specifically designed for the evaluation of the esophagus. The PillCam-ESO has the same size and shape as the small bowel capsule, but it has 2 CMOS (complementary metal oxide semiconductor) imagers, 1 at each end, which capture 7 frames per second, and it has a battery life of 20 minutes. This capsule, easily swallowed with a sip of water, is propelled through the esophagus by means of gravity and peristalsis. To slow down the esophageal transit and to decrease the presence of bubbles and/or saliva, a specific ingestion protocol has been designed. This protocol requires placing the patient on a bed with a top can be tilted to different inclinations following a strict time schedule.[43] The original ingestion protocol worked well in the initial studies. However, it gave mixed results in routine application, possibly related to deviation from the protocol because of the inconvenience of capsule ingestion in the supine position. Therefore, a simplified ingestion procedure was devised in which the patient lies on a right lateral decubitus position throughout the procedure and sips 10 mL of water every 30 seconds with a straw.[44] A study comparing the 2 ingestion procedures has shown that, despite faster esophageal transit time with the simplified ingestion procedure, the visualization of the gastroesophageal junction and the completeness of visualization of the Z line are significantly better. In addition, with this new protocol, the amount of bubbles or saliva, potentially impairing visualization, is significantly decreased. Recently, a new esophageal capsule (Pillcam-ESO2)[8] with improved characteristics has also been marketed. This new capsule captures 9 frames per second for each camera and has an improved optical system (3 lenses instead of 1 with an angle of view of 156° instead of 140° and an automatic light control system). All studies published so far, however, were performed with the first generation capsule and the original ingestion procedure.

ESOPHAGEAL CAPSULE ENDOSCOPY FOR THE DETECTION OF VARICES AND PHG

Six[45–50] original studies specifically evaluating patients with esophageal varices have been published in full. In addition, some abstracts[51–53] and a few case series that included 1 to 3 patients with esophageal varices have been published.[54,55] Therefore, about 630 patients have so far undergone esophageal capsule endoscopy for the detection of esophageal varices in these studies. The performance of the esophageal capsule in identifying esophageal varices was extremely variable (**Table 1**). Using EGD as the gold standard, the sensitivity of esophageal capsule endoscopy ranged between 68% and 100%,[45,48] and the specificity between 8% and 100%.[46,53] Thus, the positive and negative predictive values showed great variability (from 69% to 100%[45,48] and from 14% to 100%,[45,50] respectively).

In the effort to evaluate the performance of esophageal capsule endoscopy in as large a population as possible, a meta-analysis[56] has been recently published that pooled most of the available papers (6 studies; 4 published in full and 2 in abstract form). The pooled estimated sensitivity of capsule endoscopy in identifying the presence of esophageal varices was 85% (95% confidence interval [CI] 80.5%–90.1%) and the specificity was 80.5% (95% CI 74.7%–85.5%). However, both these estimates showed a significant heterogeneity between the studies included. Several reasons can explain this heterogeneity. Most studies were of small size, there were differences in the definition and grading of varices, and in the underlying disease causing portal hypertension. For these reasons, the results of the meta-analysis have to be interpreted with caution.

When the authors of the meta-analysis focused their attention on patients undergoing esophageal capsule endoscopy for screening purposes (ie, patients with a recent diagnosis of liver disease undergoing gastroscopy to diagnose the presence

Table 1
Performance of esophageal capsule endoscopy in identifying esophageal varices

Author (Year)	No. of Patients	Sensitivity (%)	Specificity (%)	PPV (%)	NPV (%)	LR+	LR−
Eisen et al (2006)[45]	32	100	89	96	100	9.1	0.01
Lapalus et al (2006)[46]	21	81	100	100	57	8.75	0.19
Smith et al (2007; abstract)[51]	15	100	67	NA	NA	3.03	0.01
Groce et al (2007; abstract)[52]	21	78	83	78	83	4.6	0.26
Pena et al (2008)[50]	20	68	100	100	14	6.8	0.32
Jensen et al (2008; abstract)[53]	50	79	8	NA	NA	NA	NA
de Franchis et al (2008)[47]	288	84	88	92	77	7.0	0.18
Lapalus et al (2009)[49]	120	77	86	69	90	5.5	0.26

Abbreviations: LR, likelihood ratio; NA, not available; NPV, negative predictive value; PPV, positive predictive value.

of varices and/or PHG), they found good sensitivity (pooled estimated sensitivity 82.7%; 95% CI 72.2%–90.4%), but specificity was low (pooled estimated specificity 54.8%; 95% CI 36.0%–72.7%) with capsule endoscopy and there was significant heterogeneity among studies. The results of a recently published French study,[49] including 120 patients undergoing esophageal capsule endoscopy for screening, closely match those of the largest published study (including more than 280 patients), which was included in the meta-analysis.[47]

The international guidelines[16–21] supporting endoscopic screening/surveillance programs for cirrhotic patients with portal hypertension pointed out that the estimation of variceal size is the key item in deciding the timing for further examinations and treatment. To reach this goal, several attempts have been made to establish an easy, reliable, and effective scoring system with conventional endoscopy. Even though different grading systems for conventional endoscopy still exist, they are all are consistently based on the persistence of linear or tortuous varices in the distal esophagus despite a complete distension of the viscus by means of forced insufflation. Unfortunately, esophageal capsule endoscopy has no insufflation. Therefore the existing grading systems for EGD cannot be transferred from traditional endoscopy to esophageal capsule endoscopy. A brand new grading system for capsule endoscopy, based on the percentage of the circumference of the capsule picture frame occupied by the largest varix, has been tested in an international multicenter study (**Fig. 3**).[47] In this study, varices were labeled as small when less than a quadrant of the circumference was occupied, and as large when 1 varix occupied more than that. Thus large varices were deemed eligible for treatment. Following this grading system, the investigators described a substantial concordance between esophageal capsule endoscopy and EGD with 91% overall agreement, a k value of 0.76 (indicating good agreement between the 2 techniques), sensitivity of 78%, and specificity of 96%. More recently 2 other studies,[48,49] using different grading systems, reproduced similar results (**Table 2**). These studies suggested that grading is possible using esophageal capsule endoscopy, but further studies are necessary to identify the best method of grading using capsule endoscopy.

For PHG, when esophageal capsule endoscopy is compared with EGD,[45,47–49] the sensitivity and specificity vary greatly (from 74% to 100% and from 17% to 83%, respectively) (**Table 3**).

Based on these data, could esophageal capsule endoscopy be proposed as a valid alternative to EGD for patients with portal hypertension? To answer this question, many factors have to be considered. The performance of the esophageal capsule

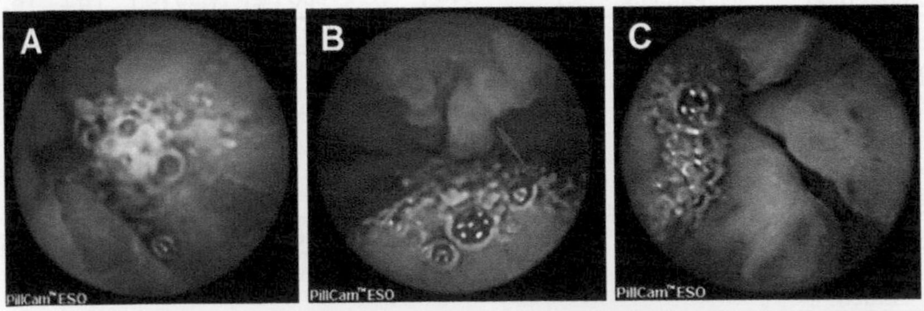

Fig. 3. Grading system for esophageal varices proposed by de Franchis and colleagues.[47] (*A*) normal Z line; (*B*) small varices occupying less than 25% of the capsule picture frame; (*C*) large varices occupying more than 25% of the capsule picture frame. (*Data from* Lapalus MG, Dumortier J, Fumex F, et al. Esophageal capsule endoscopy versus esophagogastroduodenoscopy for evaluating portal hypertension: a prospective comparative study of performance and tolerance. Endoscopy 2006;38:36–41.)

Table 2
Performance of esophageal capsule endoscopy in recognizing varices suitable for treatment

	No. of Patients	Agreement (%)	Sensitivity (%)	Specificity (%)	LR+	LR−
de Franchis et al (2008)[47]	288	91	78	96	19.5	0.2
Frenette et al (2008)[48]	50	74	63	82	3.5	2.2
Lapalus et al (2009)[49]	120	85	77	88	6.7	0.2

varies greatly across studies, and its sensitivity and specificity have to be determined in large well-selected populations, using predefined methods to grade varices at EGD as well as capsule endoscopy. In addition, a severity score for PHG at capsule endoscopy is also needed. Other issues that have to be taken into account are patient's acceptance, costs, and technical limitations of esophageal capsule endoscopy.

The less invasiveness of the capsule is 1 of the major advantages of this technique and might potentially increase the acceptance of this device for screening/surveillance programs. Nevertheless, although several studies reported that patients generally prefer capsule endoscopy over conventional EGD,[45–50] a recent paper[57] comparing esophageal capsule endoscopy, sedated EGD, and unsedated EGD performed with an ultrathin endoscope showed that the gain of capsule endoscopy over the other 2 techniques can be less relevant than expected. Although in this study, the capsule was better tolerated and accepted by patients, the investigators found that the general attitude of the patients was excellent for all 3 techniques and thus the observed advantage of capsule endoscopy is probably more of a statistical finding than a real clinical benefit. In addition, in some other studies, the investigators reported that up to 20% of patients had difficulties in swallowing the capsule in the supine position.[48]

Another major issue concerning the use of esophageal capsule endoscopy is the cost of this technique. Although programs based on esophageal capsule endoscopy may have an acceptable budgetary impact, they are highly sensitive to local costs of EGD and capsule endoscopy as shown by a recent study.[58] If endoscopic band ligation was inserted into the model as a possible method for the prophylaxis of variceal bleeding, a screening strategy including esophageal capsule endoscopy became inefficient.

Esophageal capsule endoscopy has some technical limitations including the inability to inflate or aspirate fluids and the absence of steering capability. These limitations impair not only the detection of esophageal but also of gastric varices. Although some case reports showed correct identification of gastric varices by the capsule, in the study of Lapalus and colleagues,[49] the capsule correctly identified only 1 of 8 patients with gastric varices. This is understandable, because the capsule moves inside the stomach in a chaotic way, propelled by gravity and peristalsis, with the inherent risk of missing relevant gastric findings not associated with portal hypertension (such as ulcers, erosions, or gastritis). Capsule endoscopy cannot perform biopsies, which are sometimes required in patients undergoing EGD for portal hypertension.

Table 3
Performances of esophageal capsule endoscopy in identifying PHG

	N	Sensitivity (%)	Specificity (%)	LR+	LR−
de Franchis et al (2008)[47]	288	74	83	4.4	0.31
Frenette et al (2008)[48]	50	96	17	5.6	0.04
Eisen et al (2006)[45]	19	100	77	4.3	0.00
Lapalus et al (2009)[49]	120	72	61	1.8	0.46

SMALL BOWEL CAPSULE ENDOSCOPY FOR THE DETECTION OF PHG

In the last 4 years, 8 papers (3 only available in abstract form) have been published on this topic, including a total of about 250 patients.[1,59–65] The patients included in these studies were extremely heterogeneous in terms of severity, duration, and cause of the underlining disease. The main difference among these studies is the clinical indication for capsule endoscopy. In 5 out of 8 studies (including about 140 subjects), the patients with portal hypertension underwent capsule endoscopy because of a concomitant unexplained blood loss[1,62–65]; in the remaining 3 studies, the examination was performed only to document changes in the small bowel caused by portal hypertension (**Table 4**).[59–61]

For this reason it is questionable whether these studies should be considered together, but the overall prevalence of PHE reported in studies enrolling patients with concomitant anemia (62.9%; range 48%–91%) closely matched that reported in studies involving patients with normal hemoglobin values (65.7%; range 50%–82%). These findings clearly indicate that the prevalence of PHE among patients with portal hypertension is higher than previously reported in studies using conventional endoscopes, but its role in causing chronic blood loss or anemia remains uncertain. Despite this uncertainty, capsule endoscopy was able to identify the potential source of bleeding in most of these patients,[65] and in 10%–15% of cases it showed a source of active bleeding.[64,65]

In 4 studies (involving anemic and nonanemic patients),[1,60,61,64] the prevalence of PHE has been compared with similar changes observed in controls (patients without portal hypertension mostly undergoing capsule endoscopy for obscure gastrointestinal bleeding). As expected, in all these studies the frequency of mucosal changes, defined as PHE, was significantly higher in patients with portal hypertension than in controls. Some investigators evaluated the possible correlation between the presence of PHE, documented by capsule endoscopy, and other parameters (such as the cause of cirrhosis, Child-Pugh class, presence of PHG, size of esophageal varices, demographic data, and so forth).[1,62,64,65] The results of these correlations are remarkably conflicting across studies. Recently, Riccioni and colleagues[62] evaluated the severity of portal hypertension (by measuring HVPG in patients with cirrhosis undergoing capsule endoscopy for anemia) and the severity of PHE and did not find any significant correlation. These data indirectly suggest that, despite the association of PHE and

Table 4
Prevalence of PHE across studies

Author (Year)	No. of Patients	Frequency in Patients with PH (%)	Frequency in Controls (%)	P
Urbain et al (2008)[59]	40	50.0	NA	NA
Figueiredo et al (2008)[60]	36	69.0	3.0	<.001
Repici et al (2005; abstract)[61]	29	82.0	48	<.001
Riccioni et al (2009; abstract)[62]	12	91.0	NA	NA
Jacob et al (2005; abstract)[63]	40	48.0	NA	NA
De Palma et al (2005)[64]	37	67.5	0.0	<.001
Canlas et al (2006)[65]	19	63.1	NA	NA

portal hypertension, the mechanisms leading to the development of these mucosal changes are likely to be multifactorial and not well understood.

SUMMARY

Since the introduction of small bowel capsule endoscopy, and more recently of esophageal capsule endoscopy, these diagnostic tools have become available for the evaluation of the consequences of portal hypertension in the esophagus, stomach, and small intestine. The main advantage of the esophageal and the small bowel capsule is the relatively less invasiveness that could potentially increase patients' adherence to endoscopic screening/surveillance programs. When esophageal capsule endoscopy was compared with traditional gastroscopy, it showed good sensitivity and specificity in recognizing the presence and the size of esophageal varices. However, the results are not consistent among studies, and more data are needed. Considering other issues such as costs, the absence of a reliable score for grading variceal size and its technical limitations at the present time, esophageal capsule endoscopy can only be recommended in patients unable or unwilling to undergo traditional EGD. Capsule endoscopy is safe and with continued innovations in this field, it could potentially become an alternative to traditional EGD.

As far as small bowel capsule endoscopy is concerned, the use of this device in portal hypertension showed a prevalence of mucosal changes higher than previously reported, but its clinical relevance remains undefined. Based on our current understanding, the indication for small bowel capsule endoscopy in patients with portal hypertension and concomitant anemia is to identify any source of bleeding.

REFERENCES

1. Goulas S, Triantafyllidou K, Karagiannis S, et al. Capsule endoscopy in the investigation of patients with portal hypertension and anemia. Can J Gastroenterol 2008;22(5):469–74.
2. Sanyal AJ, Bosch J, Blei A, et al. Portal hypertension and its complications. Gastroenterology 2008;134(6):1715–28.
3. Ripoll C, Groszmann R, Garcia-Tsao G, et al. Hepatic venous pressure gradient predicts clinical decompensation in patients with compensated cirrhosis. Gastroenterology 2007;133:481–8.
4. Digestive disease in the United States: epidemiology and impact. Bethesda (MD): NIDDK; 1994. NIH Publication No. 94–1447. Available at: http://digestive.niddk.nih.gov/statistics/statistics.htm. Accessed March 24, 2010.
5. Collins JG. Prevalence of selected chronic conditions: United States, 1990–1992. National Center for Health Statistics. Vital Health Stat 1997;10(194):1–89.
6. Schuppan D, Afdhal NH. Liver cirrhosis. Lancet 2008;371(9615):838–51.
7. Cichoz-Lach H, Celinski K, Slomka M, et al. Pathophysiology of portal hypertension. J Physiol Pharmacol 2008;59(Suppl 2):231–8.
8. Vianna A, Hayes PC, Moscoso G, et al. Normal venus circulation of the gastroesophageal junction. A route to understanding varices. Gastroenterology 1987; 93:876–89.
9. de Franchis R. Non-invasive (and minimally invasive) diagnosis of oesophageal varices. J Hepatol 2008;49:520–7.
10. D'Amico G, Garcia-Tsao G, Pagliaro L. Natural history and prognostic indicators of survival in cirrhosis: a systematic review of 118 studies. J Hepatol 2006;44:217–31.

11. D'Amico G, de Franchis R, a cooperative study group. Upper digestive bleeding in cirrhosis: post-therapheutic outcomes and prognostic indicators. Hepatology 2003;38:599–612.
12. Chalasani N, Kahi C, Francois S, et al. Improved patient survival after acute variceal bleeding: a multicenter, cohort study. Am J Gastroenterol 2003; 98:653–9.
13. Carbonell N, Pauwels A, Serfaty L, et al. Improved survival after variceal bleeding in patients with cirrhosis over the past two decades. Hepatology 2004;40:652–9.
14. D'Amico G, Pagliaro L, Bosch J. Pharmacologic treatment of portal hypertension: an evidence-based approach. Semin Liver Dis 1999;19:475–505.
15. Imperiale FT, Chalasani N. A meta-analysis of endoscopic variceal ligation for primary prophylaxis of oesophageal variceal bleeding. Hepatology 2001; 33:802–7.
16. de Franchis R. Developing consensus in portal hypertension. J Hepatol 1996; 25:390–4.
17. Grace ND, Groszmann RJ, Garcia-Tsao G, et al. Portal hypertension and variceal bleeding: an AASLD single topic symposium. Hepatology 1998;28:868–80.
18. Jalan R, Hayes PC. UK guidelines on the management of variceal haemorrhage in cirrhotic patients. Gut 2000;46(Suppl III):1–15.
19. de Franchis R. Updating consensus in portal hypertension. J Hepatol 2000; 33:846–52.
20. de Franchis R. Evolving consensus in portal hypertension. Report of the Baveno IV consensus workshop on methodology of diagnosis and therapy in portal hypertension. J Hepatol 2005;43:167–76.
21. Garcia-Tsao G, Sanyal AJ, Grace ND, et al. Prevention and management of gastrooesophageal varices and variceal hemorrhage in cirrhosis. Hepatology 2007; 46:922–38.
22. McCormack TT, Sims J, Eire-Brook I, et al. Gastric lesions in portal hypertension: inflammatory gastritis or congestive gastropathy? Gut 1985;26:1226–32.
23. Carpinelli L, Primignani M, Preatoni P, et al. Portal hypertensive gastropathy: reproducibility of a classification, prevalence of elementary lesions, sensitivity and specificity in the diagnosis of cirrhosis of the liver. Ital J Gastroenterol Hepatol 1997;29(6):533–40.
24. Primignani M, Carpinelli L, Preatoni P, et al. Natural history of portal hypertensive gastropathy in patients with liver cirrhosis. The New Italian Endoscopic Club for the study and treatment of esophageal varices (NIEC). Gastroenterology 2000; 119(1):181–7.
25. Iwao T, Toyonaga A, Oho K, et al. Portal-hypertensive gastropathy develops less in patients with cirrhosis and fundal varices. J Hepatol 1997;26:1235–41.
26. Thuluvath PJ, Yoo HY. Portal hypertensive gastropathy. Am J Gastroenterol 2002; 97:2973–8.
27. Tarnawski AS, Sarfeh IJ, Stachura J, et al. Microvascular abnormalities of the portal hypertensive gastric mucosa. Hepatology 1988;8(6):1488–94.
28. Sarfeh IJ, Tarnawaski A. Gastric mucosal vasculopathy in portal hypertension. Gastroenterology 1987;93:1129–31.
29. Spina GP, Arcidiacono R, Bosch J, et al. Gastric endoscopic features in portal hypertension: final report of a consensus conference, Milan, Italy, September 19, 1992. J Hepatol 1994;21:461–7.
30. Yoo HY, Eustace JA, Verma S, et al. Accuracy and reliability of the endoscopic classification of portal hypertensive gastropathy. Gastrointest Endosc 2002; 56:675–80.

31. Cales P, Zabotto B, Meskens C, et al. Gastroesophageal endoscopic features in cirrhosis. Observer variability, interassociations, and relationship to hepatic dysfunction. Gastroenterology 1990;98:156–62.
32. Burak KW, Beck PL. Diagnosis of portal hypertensive gastropathy. Curr Opin Gastroenterol 2003;19:477–82.
33. Higaki N, Matsui H, Imaoka H, et al. Characteristic endoscopic features of portal hypertensive enteropathy. J Gastroenterol 2008;43(5):327–31.
34. Barakat M, Mostafa M, Mahran Z, et al. Portal hypertensive duodenopathy: clinical, endoscopic, and histopathologic profiles. Am J Gastroenterol 2007; 102:2793–802.
35. Kodama M, Uto H, Numata M, et al. Endoscopic characterization of the small bowel in patients with portal hypertension evaluated by double balloon endoscopy. J Gastroenterol 2008;43:589–96.
36. Rondonotti E, Villa F, Signorelli C, et al. Portal hypertensive enteropathy. Gastrointest Endosc Clin N Am 2006;16:277–86.
37. Misra SP, Dwivedi M, Misra V, et al. Ileal varices and portal hypertensive ileopathy in patients with cirrhosis and portal hypertension. Gastrointest Endosc 2004; 60:778–83.
38. Desai N, Desai D, Pethe V, et al. Portal hypertensive jejunopathy: a case control study. Indian J Gastroenterol 2004;23:99–101.
39. Iddan GJ, Swain CP. History and development of capsule endoscopy. Gastrointest Endosc Clin N Am 2004;14:1–9.
40. Ramirez FC, Hakim S, Tharalson E, et al. Feasibility and safety of string wireless capsule endoscopy in the diagnosis of esophageal varices. Am J Gastroenterol 2005;100:1065–71.
41. Ramirez FC, Akins R, Shaukat M. Screening of Barrett's esophagus with string-capsule endoscopy: a prospective blinded study of 100 consecutive patients using histology as the criterion standard. Gastrointest Endosc 2008;68:25–31.
42. Liao Z, Gao R, Xu C, et al. Sleeve string capsule endoscopy for real-time viewing of the esophagus: a pilot study (with video). Gastrointest Endosc 2009;70:201–9.
43. Eliakim R, Yassin K, Shlomi I, et al. A novel diagnostic tool for detecting esophageal pathology: the PillCam oesophageal video capsule. Aliment Pharmacol Ther 2004;20(7):1083–9.
44. Gralnek IM, Rabinowitz R, Afik D, et al. A simplified ingestion procedure for esophageal capsule endoscopy: initial evaluation in healthy volunteers. Endoscopy 2006;38:913–8.
45. Eisen GM, Eliakim R, Zaman A, et al. The accuracy of PillCam ESO capsule endoscopy versus conventional upper endoscopy for the diagnosis of esophageal varices: a prospective three-center pilot study. Endoscopy 2006;38:31–5.
46. Lapalus MG, Dumortier J, Fumex F, et al. Esophageal capsule endoscopy versus esophagogastroduodenoscopy for evaluating portal hypertension: a prospective comparative study of performance and tolerance. Endoscopy 2006;38:36–41.
47. de Franchis R, Eisen GM, Laine L, et al. Esophageal capsule endoscopy for screening and surveillance of esophageal varices in patients with portal hypertension. Hepatology 2008;47:1595–603.
48. Frenette CT, Kuldau JG, Hillebrand DJ, et al. Comparison of esophageal capsule endoscopy and esophagogastroduodenoscopy for diagnosis of esophageal varices. World J Gastroenterol 2008;14(28):4480–5.

49. Lapalus MG, Ben Sousan E, Gaudric M, et al. Esophageal capsule endoscopy vs. EGD for the evaluation of portal hypertension: a French prospective multicenter comparative study. Am J Gastroenterol 2009;104(5):1112–8.
50. Pena LR, Cox T, Koch AG, et al. Study comparing oesophageal capsule endoscopy versus EGD in the detection of varices. Dig Liver Dis 2008;40:216–23.
51. Smith BW, Jeffrey GP, Adams LA, et al. Utilisation of capsule endoscopy in variceal screening and surveillance. J Gastroenterol Hepatol 2007;22:A343.
52. Groce JR, Raju GS, Sood GK, et al. A prospective single blinded comparative trial of capsule esophagoscopy vs. traditional EGD for variceal screening [abstract]. Gastroenterology 2007;132(Suppl 2):A802.
53. Jensen DM, Singh B, Chavalitdhamrong D, et al. Is capsule endoscopy accurate enough to screen cirrhotics for high risk varices & other lesions? A blinded comparison of EGD & PillCam ESO. Gastrointest Endosc 2008;67:AB122.
54. Delvaux M, Papanikolaou IS, Fassler I, et al. Esophageal capsule endoscopy in patients with suspected esophageal disease: double blinded comparison with esophagogastroduodenoscopy and assessment of interobserver variability. Endoscopy 2008;40:16–22.
55. Sanchez-Yague A, Caunedo-Alvarez A, Garcia-Montes JM, et al. Esophageal capsule endoscopy in patients refusing conventional endoscopy for the study of suspected esophageal pathology. Eur J Gastroenterol Hepatol 2006; 18:977–83.
56. Lu Y, Gao R, Liao Z, et al. Meta-analysis of capsule endoscopy in patients diagnosed or suspected with esophageal varices. World J Gastroenterol 2009; 15(10):1254–8.
57. Nakos G, Karagiannis S, Ballas S, et al. A study comparing tolerability, satisfaction and acceptance of three different techniques for esophageal endoscopy: sedated conventional, unsedated peroral ultra thin, and esophageal capsule. Dis Esophagus 2009;22:447–52.
58. Spiegel BMR, Esrailian E, Eisen G. The budget impact of endoscopic screening for esophageal varices in cirrhosis. Gastrointest Endosc 2007;66(4):679–92.
59. Urbain D, Vandebosch S, Hindryckx P, et al. Capsule endoscopy findings in cirrhosis with portal hypertension: a prospective study. Dig Liver Dis 2008; 40:391–3.
60. Figueiredo P, Almeida N, Lerias C, et al. Effect of portal hypertension in the small bowel: an endoscopic approach. Dig Dis Sci 2008;53:2144–50.
61. Repici A, Pennazio M, Ottobrelli A, et al. Endoscopic capsule in cirrhotic patients with portal hypertension: spectrum and prevalence of small bowel lesions. Endoscopy 2005;37(Suppl 1):A72.
62. Riccioni ME, Annicchiarico B, Di Stasi C, et al. Portal hypertension severity does not predict capsule endoscopy findings in the small bowel of patients with liver cirrhosis and chronic anemia. Dig Liver Dis 2009;41S:S1–67.
63. Jacob P, Favre O, Daudet J, et al. Clinical impact of capsule endoscopy for unexplained bleeding in cirrhosis; results from 21 patients. Endoscopy 2005;37(Suppl 1):A287.
64. De Palma G, Rega M, Masone S, et al. Mucosal abnormalities in patients with cirrhosis and portal hypertension: a capsule endoscopy study. Gastrointest Endosc 2005;62:529–34.
65. Canlas KR, Dobozi BM, Lin S, et al. Using capsule endoscopy to identify GI tract lesions in cirrhotic patients with portal hypertension and chronic anemia. J Clin Gastroenterol 2008;42:844–8.

Endoscopic Ultrasonography for the Evaluation of Portal Hypertension

Angels Ginès, MD, PhD*, Glòria Fernández-Esparrach, MD, PhD

KEYWORDS

• Endoscopic ultrasonography • Portal hypertension
• Vascular anatomy

Since the 1980s, endoscopic ultrasonography (EUS) has been useful in the evaluation of portal hypertension, either for the diagnostic aspects or for the evaluation of therapy and risk of bleeding. More recently, it has been described as a method for guiding interventions such as variceal injection, portal vein catheterization, or even for creating an intrahepatic portosystemic shunt in the animal laboratory.

For several years, the linear-array scanning echoendoscope was the only scope equipped with a color Doppler system. However, the new generation of radial electronic echoendoscopes is equipped with color Doppler capability too, allowing for measurement of any hemodynamic parameter of the portal circulation.

This article summarizes the current knowledge on the role of EUS for the evaluation of portal hypertension.

RECOGNITION OF INTRAMURAL VASCULAR CHANGES IN PORTAL HYPERTENSION

EUS is a good technique for visualizing vascular changes within the esophageal, gastric, and rectal walls in patients with portal hypertension (**Box 1**).[1] Esophageal varices are visualized as rounded anechoic structures just beneath the mucosal and submucosal layers (**Fig. 1**). Gastric varices are seen on EUS as anechoic serpiginous structures within the gastric wall, mainly in the fundus or at the cardia, below the esophagogastric junction (**Fig. 2**). Perforating veins are seen as serpiginous echo-free tubular structures, usually of smaller diameter than varices, going from outside the wall to the submucosa through the muscularis propria (**Fig. 3**) and connecting paraesophagogastric collateral veins with luminal gastroesophageal varices. Gastropathy appears as numerous rounded echo-free structures within the submucosa of the stomach (**Fig. 4**).

Endoscopy Unit, Institut de Malalties Digestives i Metabòliques, Hospital Clínic, CIBERehd, IDIBAPS, University of Barcelona, Villarroel 170, Barcelona 08036, Spain
* Corresponding author.
E-mail address: magines@clinic.ub.es

Clin Liver Dis 14 (2010) 221–229
doi:10.1016/j.cld.2010.03.005
liver.theclinics.com

Box 1
EUS findings in portal hypertension

Dilation of portal, splenic, and azygos veins

Dilation of the thoracic duct

Presence of:

- Periesophageal collateral veins
- Paraesophageal collateral veins
- Perigastric collateral veins
- Paragastric collateral veins
- Intramural veins (inside the muscularis propria)
- Perforating veins

Thickness of gastric mucosa and submucosa layers

Caletti and colleagues[2] compared vascular findings in 40 patients with portal hypertension with those in 48 control subjects. EUS did not display esophageal or gastric varices, periesophageal collaterals, or portal hypertensive gastropathy in control subjects, whereas the azygos, splenic, mesenteric, and portal veins were seen in both patients and controls. EUS was significantly inferior to upper endoscopy in detecting and grading esophageal varices, but superior in displaying gastric varices. Detection of periesophageal veins increased with the diameter of the varices (57%, 89%, and 100% in grades 1, 2, and 3, respectively), as well as the diameter of the azygos vein. In this study, the presence of gastric varices did not correlate with any other finding. In another study, EUS findings were compared with upper endoscopy in 58 patients with portal hypertension and controls.[3] Esophageal, gastric, periesophageal and perigastric varices, perforating veins, dilation of portal, splenic, upper mesenteric, and azygos veins, and the thoracic duct were seen in a high percentage of patients, but none of these changes was observed in controls. In this study, the assessment of gastric varices was superior with EUS than with upper endoscopy. Upper endoscopy, however, was more sensitive than EUS in detecting and grading esophageal varices. Esophageal wall compression by the balloon of the echoendoscope or the close proximity of the tip of the echoendoscope to the esophageal

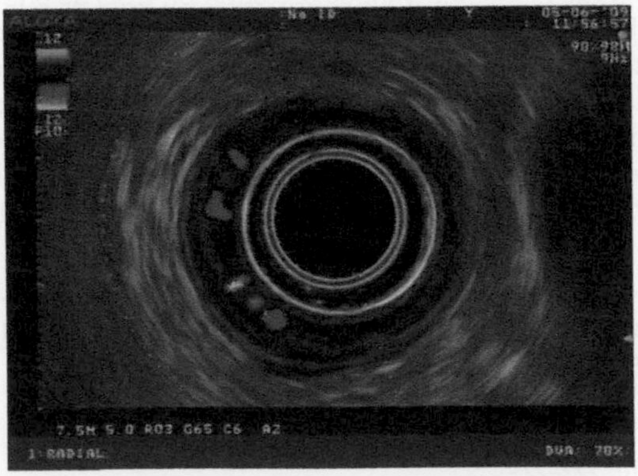

Fig. 1. Esophageal varices inside the esophageal wall, which are highlighted by the use of color Doppler.

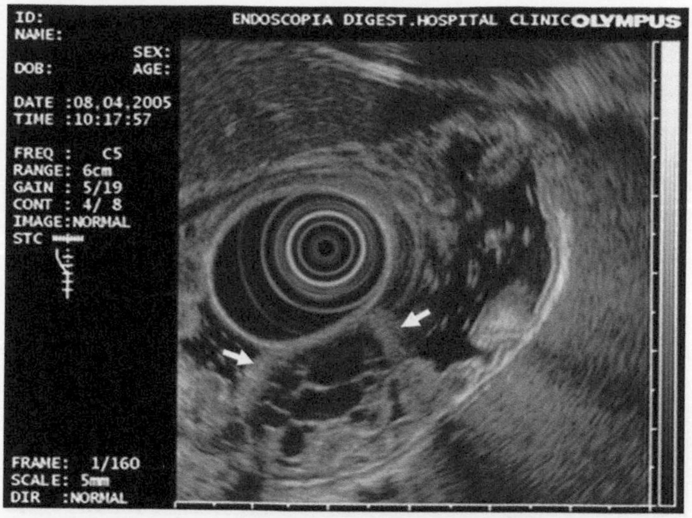

Fig. 2. Gastric varices seen as round anechoic structures inside the gastric wall (*arrows*).

wall, which is not within the focal zone of the transducer, may explain these observations. Similar observations have been made by other investigators.[4] The visualization of the esophageal varices may improve by using high-frequency miniprobes, as demonstrated in several studies.[5,6]

The diagnosis of gastric varices is probably the most important clinical indication of EUS in patients with portal hypertension. Several studies have demonstrated that EUS is superior to upper endoscopy in identifying gastric varices.[2,3,7–10] EUS may be able to differentiate between enlarged gastric folds and gastric varices. Similarly, in the rectum EUS is able to identify colorectal varices and congestive rectopathy in patients with portal hypertension.[11] EUS may also be useful for the evaluation of intramural vessels of uncommon locations, such as duodenal varices.[12,13]

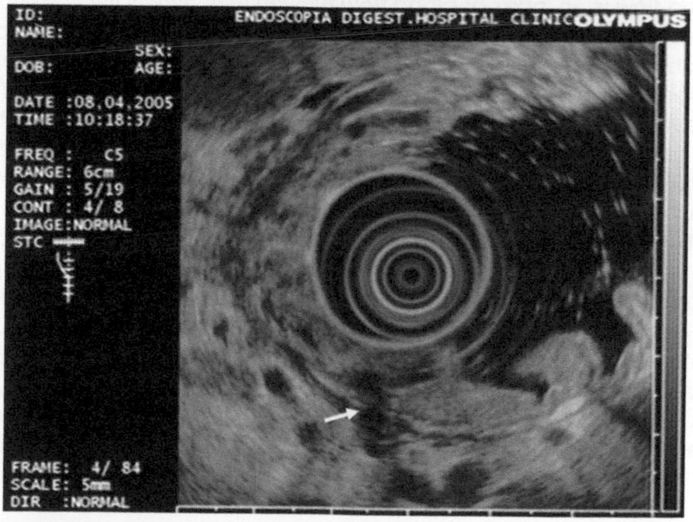

Fig. 3. Perforating vein going from the surrounding gastric tissue to the submucosal layer of the wall (*arrow*).

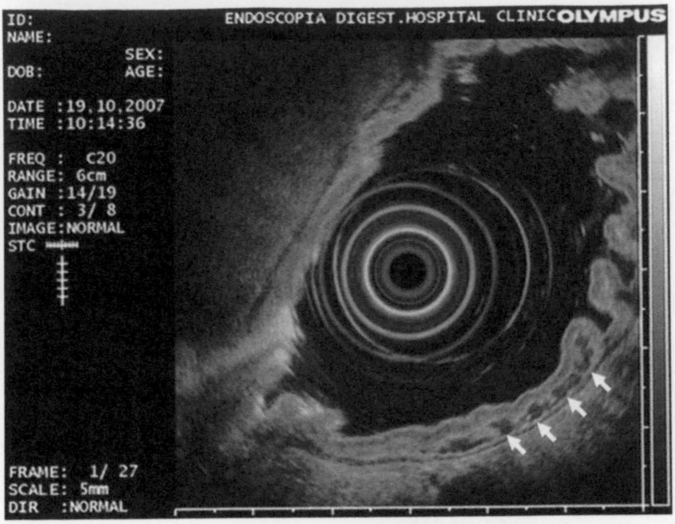

Fig. 4. Hypertensive gastropathy consisting in multiple small vessels inside the gastric wall (*arrows*).

RECOGNITION OF VASCULAR ABNORMALITIES OUTSIDE THE GASTROINTESTINAL WALL

EUS is a reliable tool in patients with portal hypertension for assessment of collaterals, the azygos vein, and the thoracic duct. These vascular structures, which cannot be assessed by upper endoscopy, play a crucial role in important clinical events in patients with portal hypertension, such as risk of rebleeding.

The azygos vein, which is easy to identify also in normal subjects, appears as a round and anechoic structure between the esophageal wall, the aorta and the spine. Its arch is easily seen adjacent to the right part of the esophageal wall. It is known that azygos blood flow is an index of blood flow through esophageal varices and collateral vessels. In fact, azygos vein dilation is common in patients with portal hypertension due to the shunting of a major portion of blood from the portal to the systemic circulation through the esophageal collateral blood vessels, which then drain into the superior vena cava via the azygos vein. Azygos flow has been known to correlate with the severity of portal hypertension, and may be used as a tool to indirectly assess the severity of portal hypertension and also to monitor the response to treatment.

Collateral vessels in the periesophageal and perigastric areas are easily seen by EUS.[14–16] Two types of collaterals have been described: periesophageal collaterals, defined as veins that are situated in the connective tissue around the esophagus or that directly make contact with the muscularis propria, and paraesophageal collaterals, which are those that do not make contact with the muscularis propria or run longitudinally distal to or over the esophagus.[17] The same applies for perigastric and paragastric collaterals. As expected, as variceal diameter increases, collateral vessels usually increase in number and diameter.[2] It has been shown that large paraesophageal and paragastric varices may be a risk factor for variceal hemorrhage.[16] In addition, the size of paraesophageal varices may be a reflection of the severity of liver failure and the presence of ascites.

A dilated thoracic duct may be identified by EUS in the posterior mediastinum, adjacent to the azygos vein, in the majority of patients with portal hypertension.[18]

ASSESSMENT OF GASTRIC MUCOSAL CHANGES

Superficial gastric layers may display some abnormalities typical of portal hypertension. Besides hypertensive gastropathy, gastric mucosa and submucosal layers are often thickened in patients with portal hypertension, most likely because of relative outflow obstruction of venous and lymphatic flow.[19]

STUDY OF HEMODYNAMIC ABNORMALITIES IN PORTAL HYPERTENSION

Although EUS is not a routine procedure in clinical practice in patients with portal hypertension, it allows for a noninvasive evaluation of the hemodynamic changes linked to this condition. Kassem and colleagues[20] demonstrated that EUS and Doppler EUS are useful to detect the hemodynamic changes in the azygos vein after variceal obliteration by endoscopic injection sclerotherapy. These investigators studied 40 patients with portal hypertension and bleeding varices who had injection sclerotherapy. The study assessed azygos vein diameter, maximal velocity, and blood flow volume index as measured by Doppler EUS before and 1 week after variceal obliteration, and found a significant increase in azygos vein diameter and blood flow volume index. This technique has been validated with reference to the standard invasive techniques to test hemodynamic changes in cirrhotic patients with portal hypertension after administration of pharmacologic agents such as somatostatin or octreotide.[21] In this study, color Doppler EUS was used to assess rapid changes in azygos blood flow after administration of placebo, somatostatin, or octreotide in a random and blinded manner, and the study confirmed the transient effects of these drugs on azygos blood flow and gastric mucosal perfusion.

In another study, 18 patients with portal hypertension were randomly selected to receive a bolus injection of terlipressin, somatostatin, or saline (controls).[22] Azygos blood flow was measured by color Doppler endosonography before and 5 and 10 minutes after the administration of the vasoactive agents or placebo. This study also concluded that Doppler EUS is a useful technique for monitoring the effects of vasoactive agents.

ASSESSMENT OF RISK FACTORS FOR VARICEAL BLEEDING, VARICEAL RECURRENCE, AND REBLEEDING AFTER TREATMENT

Lo and colleagues[8] showed that EUS is a reliable technique to assess paraesophageal veins after sclerotherapy or ligation. These investigators studied 2 groups of patients with esophageal variceal bleeding treated with ligation (n = 44) or sclerotherapy (n = 35). The prevalence of paraesophageal veins was 86% in the ligation group and 51% in the sclerotherapy group. Esophageal varices recurred in 70% and 43% in the ligation and injection group, respectively and, moreover, patients in both groups with more severe paraesophageal varices had a significantly higher rate of variceal recurrence. The rate of recurrent bleeding was also significantly higher in patients with paraesophageal varices.. A possible explanation for the results could be that ligation only affects the varices in the mucosal and submucosal layers, leaving the perforating veins untouched. By contrast, sclerotherapy may be able to obliterate the perforating and the feeding veins.[23,24] Based on these studies, it has been suggested that a closer follow-up and retreatment may be needed in patients with prominent paraesophageal veins. With EUS, it is possible to evaluate successful endoscopic sclerotherapy by demonstrating a reduction in the number and size of paraesophageal collateral vessels and the disappearance of perforating veins.[25] In a study aimed at investigating whether follow-up EUS in conjunction with endoscopy after endoscopic variceal ligation would be helpful in predicting the recurrence of bleeding from varices, Leung and colleagues[26] showed that patients with large paraesophageal varices are those at highest risk of variceal recurrence and rebleeding after endoscopic ligation. These investigators studied 40 patients, who had ligation after an episode of variceal bleeding, with EUS and gastroscopy 4 weeks after obliteration of varices and every 6 months for up to 1 year. The proportion of patients developing recurrent submucosal esophageal varices as well as recurrent bleeding was significantly higher in the group of patients presenting with large paraesophageal varices. Leung and colleagues concluded that EUS can accurately identify a subset of patients with large paraesophageal varices who are at high risk of rebleeding, and they proposed careful endoscopic monitoring in these patients.

Hino and colleagues[27] examined the hemodynamics and morphology of the left gastric vein (which is the main vessel feeding esophageal varices) by color Doppler EUS to identify factors that contributed to recurrence of varices and bleeding after endoscopic treatment. The investigators found that a low hepatofugal flow velocity in the left gastric vein trunk was the only factor associated with the efficacy of the endoscopic therapy. Moreover, the incidence of the anterior branch dominant type of the left gastric vein was significantly less in the responders to therapy. The same group validated the results in a later study with a larger sample size, and firmly concluded that an anterior branch pattern dominance of the left gastric vein at EUS as well as a rapid hepatofugal flow velocity are reliable predictors of esophageal variceal recurrence.[28] Suzuki and colleagues[6] examined the esophageal wall and periesophageal area using a high-frequency (15 or 20 MHz) miniprobe in an attempt to assess endosonographic signs for recurrence of varices after combined endoscopic treatment (endoscopic ligation and sclerotherapy). Intramural vessels (not identified by the upper endoscopy) were found in the esophagus in more than half of the cirrhotic patients, and in addition there was an increased vascular network in the fundic area. The investigators suggested that follow-up of patients with portal hypertension with both endoscopy and EUS may prevent recurrent variceal bleeding by identifying those patients who need early retreatment, and thereby improve the outcomes.

EUS MEASUREMENT OF WALL TENSION OF THE ESOPHAGEAL VARICES

There have been few attempts to measure intravariceal pressure with the help of EUS. Videogastroscope with a miniature (2 mm in diameter) pressure-sensitive capsule attached to the tip of the scope was used to estimate the variceal wall tension, an important predictor of variceal rupture, in a semiquantitative and reproducible manner. Escorsell and colleagues[29] used this technique to assess the effects of different drugs on variceal hemodynamics and to study the pathophysiology of portal hypertension.[30] Other investigators have also attempted to measure intravariceal pressure in a noninvasive manner.[31,32] At present, these promising techniques have not been validated sufficiently to apply in clinical practice.

EUS-GUIDED THERAPEUTIC INTERVENTIONS IN PORTAL HYPERTENSION

Esophageal Collateral Vessels Sclerosis

EUS has been used to guide sclerotherapy for the esophageal collateral vessels in an attempt to decrease the risk of rebleeding. In a randomized controlled trial, endoscopic sclerotherapy and EUS-guided sclerotherapy for esophageal collateral vessels were compared in 50 patients; no benefit was found with EUS-guided sclerotherapy although the recurrences tended to be less frequent and delayed in this group.[33]

Injection of Cyanocrylate in Perforating Gastric Veins

In a case series of 5 patients, EUS-guided injection of cyanoacrylate was performed in perforating veins feeding gastric varices. It was found that this technique was beneficial in eradicating the gastric varices in all patients without complications after a mean of 1.6 sessions, and moreover there was no recurrence of bleeding during 10 months of follow-up.[34] Larger comparative studies are necessary before these techniques are used in clinical practice.

EUS-Guided Portal Vein Catheterization

Among the potential clinical uses of EUS-guided portal vein catheterization, one of the most important could be the direct measurement of the portal vein pressure, if it could be done safely, in patients with portal hypertension.[35] Two feasibility studies on EUS-guided portal vein catheterization have been reported in the last year in a porcine model. Lai and colleagues[36] catheterized the extrahepatic portal vein in 85% of 14 pigs with portal hypertension and 7 controls. Pressure measurements obtained under EUS guidance showed a good correlation with those obtained by transhepatic catheterization, but one of these pigs developed severe intraperitoneal bleeding. In another study, intrahepatic portal vein was punctured with EUS guidance in 5 pigs, without any hemorrhagic complications.[37] These investigators suggested that EUS-guided portal vein catheterization is feasible, safe, and could be used for portal angiography and pressure measurements. More safety studies in portal hypertensive animals are necessary before human studies are attempted.

Recently, Buscaglia and colleagues[38] described the creation of a transjugular intrahepatic portosystemic shunt under linear-array EUS guidance. The technique was successful in 10 pigs, with no evidence of bleeding or damage to intraperitoneal organs. The investigators suggested that EUS-guided intrahepatic portosystemic shunt could be an alternative to the conventional methods of transjugular intrahepatic portosystemic shunt placement. EUS in combination with percutaneous transhepatic portography has also been used in the preoperative evaluation before selecting devascularization surgery for esophagogastric varices.[39]

SUMMARY

EUS is a good technique to explore vascular changes in portal hypertension, but currently it does not have an established role in clinical practice. The potential clinical applications are for the diagnosis of gastric varices and for the evaluation of periesophageal circulation. EUS has no role in the grading of esophageal varices. In selected cases, EUS may be of help in localizing bleeding varices in ectopic locations or in guiding endoscopic therapy. Future applications may include EUS-guided portal vein catheterization and interventions, but to date, safety data are lacking.

REFERENCES

1. El-Saadany M, Jalil S, Irisawa A, et al. EUS for portal hypertension: a comprehensive and critical appraisal of clinical and experimental indications. Endoscopy 2008;40:690–6.
2. Caletti G, Brocchi E, Baraldini M, et al. Assessment of portal hypertension by endoscopic ultrasonography. Gastrointest Endosc 1990;36:S21–7.
3. Burtin P, Calès P, Oberti F, et al. Endoscopic ultrasonographic signs of portal hypertension in cirrhosis. Gastrointest Endosc 1996;44:257–61.

4. Boustière C, Dumas O, Jouffre C, et al. Gastric endoscopic ultrasonography: a new approach to the diagnosis of portal hypertension in cirrhotic patients. Hepatology 1991;14:85.
5. Liu JB, Miller LS, Feld RI, et al. Gastric and esophageal varices: 20-MHz transnasal endoluminal US. Radiology 1993;187:363–6.
6. Suzuki T, Matsutani S, Umebara K, et al. EUS changes predictive for recurrence of esophageal varices in patients treated by combined endoscopic ligation and sclerotherapy. Gastrointest Endosc 2000;52:611–7.
7. Konishi Y, Nakamura T, Kida H, et al. Catheter US probe EUS evaluation of gastric cardia and perigastric vascular structures to predict esophageal variceal recurrence. Gastrointest Endosc 2002;55:197–203.
8. Lo GH, Lai KH, Cheng JS, et al. Prevalence of paraesophageal varices and gastric varices in patients achieving variceal obliteration by banding ligation and by injection sclerotherapy. Gastrointest Endosc 1999;49:428–36.
9. Pontes JM, Leitao MC, Portela FA, et al. Endoscopic ultrasonography in the treatment of esophageal varices by endoscopic sclerotherapy and band ligation: do we need it. Eur J Gastroenterol Hepatol 1995;7:41–6.
10. Lee YT, Chan FK, Ching JY, et al. Diagnosis of gastroesophageal varices and portal collateral venous abnormalities by endosonography in cirrhotic patients. Endoscopy 2002;34:391–8.
11. Goenka MK, Kochhar R, Nagi B, et al. Rectosigmoid varices and other mucosal changes in patients with portal hypertension. Am J Gastroenterol 1991;86:1185–9.
12. Wu CS, Chen CM, Chang KY. Endoscopic injection sclerotherapy of bleeding duodenal varices. J Gastroenterol Hepatol 1995;19:481–3.
13. Palazzo L, Hochain P, Helmer C, et al. Biliary varices on endoscopic ultrasonography: clinical presentation and outcome. Endoscopy 2000;32:520–4.
14. Sanyal AJ. The value of EUS in the management of portal hypertension. Gastrointest Endosc 2000;52:575–7.
15. Caletti GC, Brocchi E, Ferrari A, et al. Value of endoscopic ultrasonography in the management of portal hypertension. Endoscopy 1992;24(Suppl 1):342–6.
16. Faigel DO, Rosen HR, Sasaki A, et al. EUS in cirrhotic patients with and without prior variceal hemorrhage in comparison with noncirrhotic control subjects. Gastrointest Endosc 2000;52:455–62.
17. Irisawa A, Obara K, Sato Y, et al. EUS analysis of collateral veins inside and outside the esophageal wall in portal hypertension. Gastrointest Endosc 1999; 50:374–80.
18. Parasher VK, Meroni E, Malesci A, et al. Observation of thoracic duct morphology in portal hypertension by endoscopic ultrasound. Gastrointest Endosc 1998;48: 588–92.
19. Avunduk C, Hampf F. Endoscopic ultrasound in the diagnosis of watermelon stomach. J Clin Gastroenterol 1996;22:104–6.
20. Kassem AM, Salama ZA, Zakaria MS, et al. Endoscopic ultrasonography study of the azygos vein before and after endoscopic obliteration of esophagogastric varices by injection sclerotherapy. Endoscopy 2000;32:630–4.
21. Nishida H, Giostra E, Spahr L, et al. Validation of color Doppler EUS for azygos blood flow measurement in patients with cirrhosis: application to the acute hemodynamic effects of somatostatin, octreotide, or placebo. Gastrointest Endosc 2001;54:24–30.
22. Lee YT, Sung JJY, Yung MY, et al. Use of color Doppler EUS in assessing azygos blood flow for patients with portal hypertension. Gastrointest Endosc 1999;50: 47–52.

23. Nakamura H, Endo M, Shumojuu K, et al. Esophageal varices evaluated by endoscopic ultrasonography: observation of collateral circulation during non-shunting operations. Surg Endosc 1990;4:69–75.
24. Kitano S, Terblanche J, Kahn D, et al. Venous anatomy of the lower esophagus in portal hypertension: practical implications. Br J Surg 1986;73:525–31.
25. Dhiman RK, Choudhuri G, Saraswat VA, et al. Role of paraesophageal collateral and perforating veins on outcome of endoscopic sclerotherapy for esophageal varices: an endosonographic study. Gut 1996;38:759–64.
26. Leung VK, Sung JJ, Ahuja AT, et al. Large paraesophageal varices on endosonography predict recurrence of esophageal varices rebleeding. Gastroenterology 1997;112:1811–6.
27. Hino S, Kakutani H, Ikeda K, et al. Hemodynamic analysis of esophageal varices using color Doppler endoscopic ultrasonography to predict recurrence after endoscopic treatment. Endoscopy 2001;33:869–72.
28. Kuramochi A, Imazu H, Kakutani H, et al. Color Doppler endoscopic ultrasonography in identifying groups at high-risk of recurrence of esophageal varices after endoscopic treatment. J Gastroenterol 2007;42:219–24.
29. Escorsell A, Bordas JM, Feu F, et al. Endoscopic assessment of variceal volume and wall tension in cirrhotic patients: effects of pharmacological therapy. Gastroenterology 1997;113:1640–6.
30. Escorsell A, Ginès A, Llach J, et al. Increasing intra-abdominal pressure increases pressure, volume, and wall tension in esophageal varices. Hepatology 2002;36:936–40.
31. Miller ES, Kim JK, Gandehok J, et al. A new device for measuring esophageal variceal pressure. Gastrointest Endosc 2002;56:284–91.
32. Miller LS, Dai Q, Thomas A, et al. A new ultrasound-guided esophageal variceal pressure-measuring device. Am J Gastroenterol 2004;99:1267–73.
33. de Paulo GA, Ardengh JC, Nakao FS, et al. Treatment of esophageal varices: a randomized controlled trial comparing endoscopic sclerotherapy and EUS-guided sclerotherapy of esophageal collateral veins. Gastrointest Endosc 2006; 63:396–402.
34. Romero-Castro R, Pellicer-Bautista FJ, Jiménez-Saenz M, et al. EUS-guided injection of cyanoacrylate in perforating feeding veins in gastric varices: results in 5 cases. Gastrointest Endosc 2007;66:402–7.
35. Brugge WR. EUS is an important new tool for accessing the portal vein. Gastrointest Endosc 2008;67:343–4.
36. Lai L, Poneros J, Santilli J, et al. EUS-guided portal vein catheterization and pressure measurement in an animal model: a pilot study of feasibility. Gastrointest Endosc 2004;59:280–3.
37. Giday SA, Clarke JO, Buscaglia JM, et al. EUS-guided portal vein catheterization: a promising novel approach for portal angiography and portal vein pressure measurements. Gastrointest Endosc 2008;67:338–42.
38. Buscaglia JM, Dray X, Shin EJ, et al. A new alternative for a transjugular intrahepatic portosystemic shunt: EUS-guided creation of an intrahepatic portosystemic shunt. Gastrointest Endosc 2009;69:941–7.
39. Hsieh JS, Wang WM, Perng DS, et al. Modified devascularization surgery for isolated gastric varices assessed by endoscopic ultrasonography. Surg Endosc 2004;18:666–71.

Role of Endoscopy in Primary Prophylaxis for Esophageal Variceal Bleeding

Agustín Albillos, MD, PhD[a,b,*], Beatriz Peñas, MD[a],
Javier Zamora, MD, PhD[c,d]

KEYWORDS

- Cirrhosis • Portal hypertension • β-blockers
- Endoscopic variceal ligation

Cirrhosis is the leading cause of portal hypertension in the Western world. From a clinical standpoint, the most significant consequence of portal hypertension is the development of esophageal varices. Despite the many advances in the management of variceal bleeding, it remains a life-threatening complication of portal hypertension. Primary prophylaxis to prevent the first bleeding episode is therefore critically important in the management of patients with cirrhosis and esophageal varices. Endoscopy plays a paramount role to accomplish this task by identifying and staging the population at risk of bleeding and amenable to prophylactic therapy, and by erradicating the esophageal varices in selected cases.

ESOPHAGEAL VARICES FORMATION AND BLEEDING IN CIRRHOSIS

One of the most serious consequences of portal hypertension is the formation of esophagogastric varices. The appearance of varices in patients with compensated

This work was supported by grants from the Spanish Ministry of Education (no. BFU 2006-09280/BFI), the Fundación Mutua Madrileña (no. FundacionMM-2006-001), and from the Spanish Ministry of Health, Instituto de Salud Carlos III (PI051871, Ciberehd).
[a] Servicio de Gastroenterología y Hepatología, Hospital Universitario Ramón y Cajal, Universidad de Alcalá, Madrid, Spain
[b] Centro de Investigación Biomédica en Red de Enfermedades Hepáticas y Digestivas (Ciberehd), Instituto de Salud Carlos III, Madrid, Spain
[c] Servicio de Bioestadística Clínica, Hospital Universitario Ramón y Cajal, Universidad de Alcalá, Madrid, Spain
[d] Centro de Investigación Biomédica en Red Epidemiología y Salud Púbica (Ciberesp), Instituto de Salud Carlos III, Madrid, Spain
* Corresponding author. Servicio de Gastroenterología y Hepatología, Hospital Universitario Ramón y Cajal, Madrid, Carretera de Colmenar Viejo km 9,100, Madrid 28034, Spain.
E-mail address: aalbillosm@meditex.es

Clin Liver Dis 14 (2010) 231–250
doi:10.1016/j.cld.2010.03.001

cirrhosis marks the transition from clinical stage 1 of chronic liver disease, which carries a low risk of death (1% at 1 year), to stage 2, which is associated with an intermediate risk of death (3.4%/y).[1] For this change to occur, portal pressure, as estimated by the hepatic venous pressure gradient (HVPG), should increase more than 10 mm Hg (clinically significant portal hypertension).[2] Portal pressure is the leading force promoting the formation and development of varices. Patients with cirrhosis but without varices with an HVPG more than 10 mm Hg at the time of initial endoscopic screening have an approximately twofold greater risk of esophageal varices formation at 4 years compared with those with an HVPG less than 10 mm Hg.[3]

Once formed, esophageal varices tend to increase in size from small to large before they eventually rupture and bleed. The yearly rate of formation of new varices is about 5% to 10%, whereas the rate of progression from small to large varices ranges between 5% and 30% in the different studies.[3–6] Such variability is probably the result of differences in patient selection and follow-up endoscopy schedules. Liver failure, as assessed by Child-Pugh class, and, to a lesser extent, the alcoholic cause of cirrhosis, are the factors that have been most consistently associated with variceal growth. At the time of diagnosis, the prevalence of esophageal varices is 30% in patients with compensated cirrhosis and 60% in those with decompensated cirrhosis.[7]

Bleeding from esophagogastric varices marks the entry of the patient into the decompensated stage of cirrhosis. Variceal bleeding defines stage 4 of chronic liver disease, which shows the highest mortality at 1 year (57%).[1] Despite the therapeutic improvements of the last 10 years, bleeding from gastroesophageal varices is the most lethal complication of portal hypertension, with an associated mortality of 20% within 6 weeks of the bleeding episode.[8] Hence, it is important to prevent the first variceal bleeding episode by identifying patients at risk and providing them with prophylactic treatment.

ENDOSCOPY FOR PRIMARY PROPHYLAXIS OF ESOPHAGEAL VARICEAL BLEEDING

The risk of bleeding from esophagogastric varices in patients with cirrhosis varies widely (range 6%–76% at 1 year).[9] This broad range of reported risk may indicate the heterogeneity of the patient population, and therefore it is important to identify high-risk patients who would benefit most from primary prophylaxis. In this context, esophagogastroduodenostomy (EGD) plays a preeminent role in identifying candidate cirrhotic patients for prophylaxis against first variceal bleeding. EGD is the gold standard for the diagnosis of esophageal varices. Besides, endoscopy determines the size of varices and the presence of red signs, which, in addition to the severity of liver disease, are the 3 factors used for bleeding risk stratification, with size being the main determinant of bleeding, see the article by Coelho-Prabhu and Kamath elsewhere in this issue for further exploration of this topic.[9,10]

ENDOSCOPIC CLASSIFICATION AND GRADING OF ESOPHAGEAL VARICES

Several endoscopic classification schemes for esophageal varices have been published. The most detailed is that of the Japanese Research Society for Portal Hypertension based on variceal color, size, extension as measured proximally from the gastroesophageal junction, and the presence or absence of red signs (**Box 1**).[11,12] Red signs are small areas of a varix with a thin weak wall, likely due to maximum distension of the vessel prone to rupture. The Japanese classification system distinguishes between red wale markings (longitudinal dilated venules resembling whip marks), cherry-red spots, and hematocystic spots (saccular outpouches of the varix similar to an aneurysmal dilation), and the latter are related

Box 1
Classification of esophageal varices

Japanese Research Society for Portal Hypertension[11,12]

General color
- Blue varices
- White varices

Size (type)
- F1 (small and straight varices)
- F2 (enlarged tortuous varices, <one-third of the lumen of the esophagus)
- F3 (large and tortuous, more than one-third of the lumen of the esophagus)

Red color signs
- Red color signs absent
- Red wheal markings
- Cherry-red spots
- Hematocystic spot
- Diffuse redness
- Red wheal markings and cherry-red spots moderate or severe
- Red wheal markings and cherry-red spots absent or mild

Proximal extension
- Locus inferior (distal one-third of esophagus alone)
- Locus medialis
- Locus superior (extension to proximal one-third of esophagus)

Dagradi and colleagues[13]
- Grade I: varices with a diameter of less than or equal to 2 mm, disappear with esophageal lumen insufflation, sometimes only detectable on performance of the Vasalva maneuver
- Grade II: varices of similar diameter, clearly visible in the esophageal lumen during both phases of respiration
- Grade III: varices of 3 to 4 mm, prominent in the esophageal lumen, straight or tortuous
- Grade IV: varices of greater than or equal to 5 mm, tortuous, contact made with the varices in the opposite esophageal wall

Westaby and colleagues[14]
- Grade 1+: varices flush with the wall of esophagus
- Grade 2+: varices protrude no more than half way to the center of the esophageal lumen
- Grade 3+: varices protrude more than half way to the center of the esophageal lumen

The original Dagradi classification included a grade V, similar to grade IV but including red color signs.

to the highest risk of rupture. Other methods classify the size of varices into 4 or 3 grades through semiquantitative morphologic assessment (see **Box 1**), but fail to differentiate among the different red signs, simply considering their presence or absence.[13,14]

Controversy exists regarding the interobserver variability of EGD used to assess the presence and size of esophageal varices. Agreement is good (kappa index >0.5) for esophageal variceal size and presence of red signs.[15] The reproducibility of a semiquantitative grading scheme based on the appearance of esophageal varices (flattened by insufflation/confluent) is greater than a quantitative (cutoff 5 mm) grading system based on size.[16] Agreement is poor to fair for the presence of esophageal varices and grade of gastric varices (kappa indices from 0.38 to 0.52 and of 0.29, respectively). In general, the greater the variceal size, the better the agreement. Therefore, the effect of poor agreement in assessing esophageal varix presence or size on the current policy of primary prophylaxis is low, because the target population comprises patients with large (or medium-sized) varices.

RISK STRATIFICATION OF ESOPHAGEAL VARICES

Variceal size is the most important predictor of hemorrhage. The Baveno I Consensus Conference recommends simplifying the size classification as much as possible to define 2 grades, small and large, by semiquantitative morphologic description or by quantitative size determination applying a cutoff diameter of 5 mm.[17] For schemes that include intermediate grades, medium-sized varices should be considered to be large. Two years after the diagnosis of cirrhosis, the risk of bleeding is about 2% in patients with no varices, 8% in patients with small varices, and up to 30% in those with medium-large varices.[5,7,18]

Besides variceal size, other factors can be used to predict the risk of hemorrhage; the presence of red signs on varices and severity of liver disease (assessed by Child-Pugh class).[9] The use of these 3 independent, but related, variables was assessed by The North Italian Endoscopy Club (NIEC), which developed a prognostic index that is presently one of the most reliable predictors of variceal rupture. This index is based on data from a prospective study in which 321 patients with cirrhosis and esophageal varices without prior bleeding were followed. By multivariate analysis, the risk of bleeding correlated with variceal size, the presence of red signs, and Child-Pugh class. However, its prognostic efficiency is limited because some patients considered at low risk do bleed (about 10%) and the number of high-risk patients that can be identified is small. Among the possible reasons for the inaccuracy of the NIEC index are the continuous changes that occur in the predictive factors and the logistic difficulty of real-time monitoring.

A distinctive feature of the NIEC index is the large weight assigned to the coefficient of Child-Pugh class, which results in greater risks of bleeding in patients with advanced liver disease. Regression analysis and modeling of the NIEC index has revealed that the size of esophageal varices and presence of red signs are much more important than the Child-Pugh class in predicting a first variceal bleeding episode. **Table 1** provides the regression coefficients of the variables used to calculate the original and revised NIEC indices, indicating the lower weight coefficient given to the Child-Pugh class in the revised version.[10]

SCREENING POLICY: IDENTIFYING THE TARGET POPULATION

Based on current evidence, EGD screening for esophageal varices is recommended in all patients diagnosed with cirrhosis (**Table 2**). Moreover, EGD surveillance is needed during follow-up to detect newly formed large varices in patients with no varices or with small varices not receiving prophylaxis, because, once formed, varices tend to increase in size from small to large. Follow-up endoscopies are not needed in patients being treated with β-blockers. The mean annual incidence of esophageal varices is

Table 1
Regression coefficients of variables predicting first variceal bleeding included in the NIEC

Variable	NIEC[9] (n = 321)	Revised NIEC[10] (n = 627)
Size of varices	0.4365	1.12
Red signs	0.3193	0.36
Child-Pugh class	0.645	0.04

7%.[4–6,19] Based on this estimate and on the likelihood that newly formed varices will be small if detected after a short interval, expert consensus panels recommend repeat endoscopy after 2 to 3 years in patients in whom no varices were detected in the first endoscopy.[20,21] In those with small varices, the EGD should be repeated every 1 to 2 years, because varices progress in a mean of 12% of patients per year.[20] Because the factor most consistently associated with variceal progression is Child-Pugh class, EGD should be conducted once a year in patients with decompensated cirrhosis.[20,21]

There is general agreement that patients with medium-large (>5 mm) varices should receive prophylaxis against first bleeding. However, whether this should be extended to patients with small varices is debatable for the following reasons: (1) endoscopic assessment of variceal size is subjective. Small varices are those smaller than 5 mm, corresponding to grade F1 of the Japanese classification and grades 1 and 2 of the classifications that use 4 grades (see **Box 1**).[11–14] There is so much subjectivity that the Baveno IV Consensus Conference could not reach an agreement to define small and large varices.[22] (2) The bleeding risk of some subsets of patients with small varices is not unappreciable. According to the NIEC study, the estimated probability of bleeding within 1 year in patients with small varices and red signs is similar to the risk shown by patients with large varices without red signs (ranges 16–44 and 15–42, respectively). In addition, the risk of small varices bleeding in Child-Pugh class C patients is even greater than that of large varices in Child-Pugh class A patients (20% and 15%, respectively).[9] Therefore, it seems reasonable to consider for prophylactic therapy patients with small varices at high risk of bleeding: small varices with red signs or those occurring in Child-Pugh class C patients.

Table 2
Prophylaxis of first variceal bleeding in patients with cirrhosis

Clinical Situation	Treatment	Follow-up Endoscopy	Comments
No varices	None	Every 3 years	
Small varices	None	Every 2 years Every year if Child-Pugh class B/C	Long-term benefit of β-blockers not established
Small varices + red signs on varices or Child-Pugh class B/C	β-blockers	Not needed	
Large varices	Endoscopic band ligation	Every 6 months	Both therapies effective
	β-blockers	Not needed	Consider local expertise, patient preferences, and contraindications/intolerance to β-blockers

The prevalence of large esophageal varices at the time of cirrhosis diagnosis is around 15% to 25%.[7] On follow-up, 50% of patients may not have developed esophageal varices 6 years after the diagnosis of cirrhosis.[5] According to these figures, most EGD-screened patients will not have varices or will not require prophylactic therapy. However, adherence to current recommendations means they will undergo several unnecessary endoscopies. EGD is costly, unpleasant, usually requires sedation, and is associated with a small but significant risk of complications. These shortcomings have limited the inclusion of patients with cirrhosis in screening programs and there is now much interest in developing methods and models alternative to conventional upper endoscopy to predict the presence of high-risk varices. The methods the authors have evaluated so far include Doppler ultrasound–based models, transient elastography, computed tomography, and magnetic resonance, as well as the use of endoscopic videocapsules. These alternative procedures are commented on in other articles in this issue. So far, none of these techniques has been sufficiently accurate to replace EGD to assess the presence of esophageal varices.

Cost-effectiveness studies using a Markov model have suggested empirical treatment with β-blockers for all patients with cirrhosis,[23,24] or screening endoscopy for patients with compensated cirrhosis and universal β-blocker therapy for those with decompensated disease.[25] The conclusions of these studies are limited by variations in the methodology used for analysis, no consideration of adherence to prophylaxis strategy in most existing models, and applying different levels of evidence for analysis, including different estimates for bleeding risk reduction by endoscopic variceal ligation (EVL) and short time horizons for data extrapolation. Future studies should consider community-based patients, patient preferences, and updated data on the natural history of small varices. At present, endoscopic screening for varices in all patients with cirrhosis is the most suitable approach.

THERAPIES TO PREVENT THE FIRST EPISODE OF VARICEAL BLEEDING

The 2 options available for primary prophylaxis are pharmacologic and endoscopic therapy (**Fig. 1**). Pharmacologic therapy consists of nonselective β-blockers, which reduce the risk of bleeding by lowering portal pressure through a decrease in portal venous inflow. Endoscopic therapies, at present EVL, act locally and have no effect on portal pressure.

NONSELECTIVE β-BLOCKERS

Nonselective β-adrenergic blockers (propanolol or nadolol) are the pharmacologic therapy for the primary prophylaxis of variceal bleeding. In patients with cirrhosis and esophageal varices of any size, β-blockers reduce the risk of a first bleeding episode from 25% to 15% within 2 years; the absolute risk difference being −10% (95% confidence interval [CI], −16 to 5) and 10 being the number needed to treat for a benefit.[26] In patients with cirrhosis and large varices, β-blockers reduce the 2-year baseline risk of bleeding from 27% to 17%. The beneficial effect of β-blockers is observed irrespective of the cause and severity of cirrhosis, although it seems to be lower in patients with advanced liver disease or with ascites.[27] Mortality is lower in the β-blockers group compared with the control group[26] and this difference has been shown to be significant.[28]

The Hemodynamic Response to β-Blockers in Patients Without Previous Variceal Bleeding

β-blockers decrease portal pressure by reducing cardiac output (β_1 effect) and mainly, by allowing α-adrenergic–induced splanchnic vasoconstriction (β_2 effect), thereby

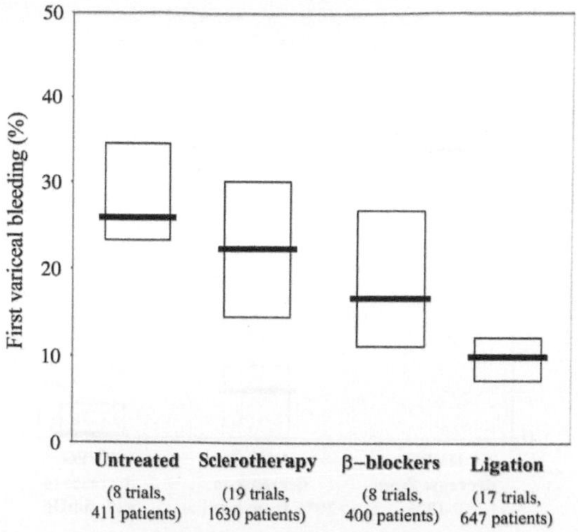

Fig. 1. Reported esophageal variceal bleeding rates in randomized trials of different treatments to prevent first variceal bleeding in patients with cirrhosis and large varices. The figure summarizes the results of studies using different treatment options included in published[26,61] and current meta-analyses. The squares represent the interquartile range and the horizontal bars the median.

reducing portal blood flow. The selective β_1-blockers (metoprolol, atenolol) are less effective for primary prophylaxis because they lack β_2 effect. To achieve protection against first bleeding, drug therapy should reduce the HVPG until a specific cutoff value. Several randomized controlled trials and prospective cohort studies have shown that a reduction in HVPG to less than 12 mm Hg virtually eliminates the risk of first variceal bleeding,[29–33] and this end point is reached in about 20% of patients on long-term β-blocker therapy.[34] A decrease in the HVPG of more than 20% from baseline is also associated with a marked reduction in the risk of first bleeding, but this target end point is reached in a greater proportion of subjects (30%).[34] Overall, β-blockers achieve either of these target end points in about 50% of patients, with bleeding recorded in 6% of responders and 32% of nonresponders (**Fig. 2**).[34,35]

The target cutoff values for HVPG mentioned earlier are commonly used in clinical trials to assess specificity. However, these cutoff values are not associated with the highest sensitivity to predict the bleeding risk. The drop in HVPG of more than 20% was defined as a cutoff during the follow-up of a cohort of patients on β-blockers to prevent variceal rebleeding.[36] This hypothesis has been tested in patients without previous bleeding when the use of less stringent criteria was found to be more sensitive for detecting responders without sacrificing specificity. A recent study has shown that the use of a cutoff value of 10% instead of 20% increases the sensitivity to detect patients with a lower risk of bleeding (responders) in the long-term from 34% to 64%.[37] The change in this criterion also improves its positive predictive value, because the rate of first bleeding among nonresponders increased from 27% to 46%. This cutoff value was also associated with a lower risk of other complications of portal hypertension, such as ascites or spontaneous bacterial peritonitis.[33,37]

Given the intimate relationship between HVPG reduction and first bleeding risk (see **Fig. 2**), an HVPG-guided primary prophylaxis strategy has been suggested. A drawback of this approach is the need to conduct 2 hemodynamic studies (at baseline and weeks after treatment) to assess the HVPG response to drug therapy. This

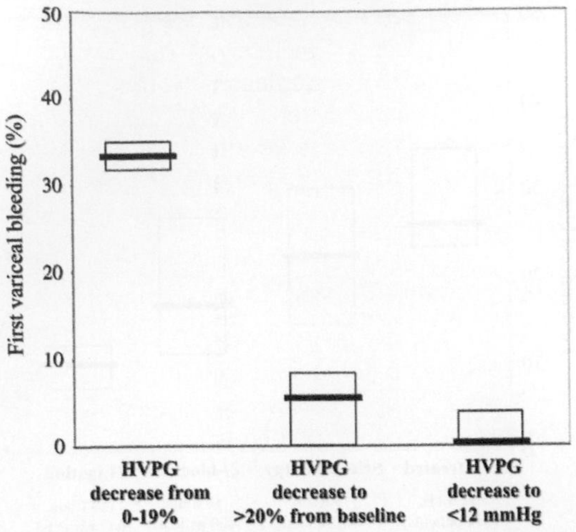

Fig. 2. Reported esophageal variceal bleeding rates in studies assessing the correlation between the HVPG response to chronic treatment with β-blockers and first variceal bleeding. The figure summarizes the results of 5 studies, 4 included in meta-analysis,[34] and a single study[37] totaling 361 patients. The squares represent the interquartile range and the horizontal bars the median.

problem has been largely overcome by the recent finding that responders to β-blockers can be identified in a single hemodynamic study, because the accuracy of using the criterion of a 10% or greater reduction in HVPG during an acute infusion to predict the HVPG response during chronic therapy is 90%.[37,38] Despite this, it is unlikely that HVPG measurements will be incorporated in the decision making for primary prophylaxis considering that (1) the positive predictive value of the 10% threshold is still low, and more than half of nonresponders do not bleed; (2) the low risk of first bleeding in patients on β-blockers; and (3) the lack of studies showing that an HVPG-guided strategy is better than current practice.

The residual risk of a first hemorrhage in patients with varices of any size on β-blockers (10% in those with varices of any size, increasing to 15% in patients with large varices) is lower than the number of nonresponders under the target HVPG end points,[26,34,35] a finding that can be explained in several ways: (1) protection from first bleeding by β-blockers needs less stringent HVPG reduction criteria than the accepted methods for the prevention of rebleeding[33,37]; or (2) the beneficial effect of β-blockers on bleeding prevention probably goes beyond their portal pressure–lowering effect. β-blockers reduce collateral blood flow, as measured by azygos blood flow (36%) and variceal pressure (~26%) to a greater extent than HVPG (~12%).[31,39,40] Reduction in azygos blood flow by β-blockers is secondary to reduction in portal venous flow and mainly to β-2-adrenoceptor blockade, and this effect is even observed in patients in whom HVPG failed to decrease beyond the target end points.[41]

Dosing β-Blockers and Side Effects

In the trials performed to date, the dose of β-blockers was determined as that producing a 25% decrease in heart rate from baseline, but this reduction does not correlate with the extent of HVPG reduction. In addition, the HVPG measurement procedure is not widely available. The current recommendation is that the dose of β-blockers should be adjusted to the maximal dose tolerated by the patient, because the β_2-blockade responsible for splanchnic vasoconstriction is more resistant than

β_1-blockade. The risk of bleeding recurs when β-blockers are stopped, thus, once initiated, β-blockade should be continued indefinitely.[42] The common adverse effects of β-blockers in patients with cirrhosis are dizziness, breathlessness, and fatigue, and these usually disappear or decrease in intensity with time or with dose adjustment. Withdrawal of β-blockers because of adverse effects is necessary in about 15% of patients.[43,44] Approximately 15% to 20% of patients are not suitable for β-blockers because of related contraindications, mainly bronchospasm, heart failure, and peripheral vascular disease.[43]

Enhancing the HPVG Response to β-Blockers Using Other Agents

Alternatives to β-blockers for primary prophylaxis are required to treat patients with contraindications or intolerance to β-blockers and to reduce the residual risk of bleeding. Drugs, such as vasodilators or diuretics, have been added to β-blockers to lower the HVPG and increase the proportion of responders. Isosorbide-5-mononitrate has an additive effect on lowering HVPG when used in combination with β-blockers, and combination treatment increases the rate of responders by about one-third.[45,46] The efficacy of β-blockers plus isosorbide-5-mononitrate has been compared in 3 trials totaling 552 patients.[47–49] Meta-analysis of these studies revealed a nonsignificant lower bleeding rate (from 15% to 10%), and greater occurrence of side effects (from 5.6% to 12%) in the combination therapy group, but mortality was similar in both groups[50]; the results remained unchanged when only patients with large varices were separately analyzed. Thus, in contrast to the secondary prophylaxis setting, in which isosorbide-5-mononitrate improved the efficacy of β-blockers, the available evidence does not support the combination of β-blockers and nitrates for primary prophylaxis. The only trial comparing the efficacy of nadolol and spironolactone with that of nadolol alone for first bleeding prophylaxis showed similar HVPG reductions, bleeding rates, and 2-year mortalities for the 2 therapeutic arms.[51]

Among the other drugs tested, angiotensin II receptor blockers have been ruled out because of their null or small portal pressure lowering effect and marked arterial hypotension produced in patients with advanced cirrhosis.[52,53] The use of isosorbide-5-mononitrate alone is not recommended because it can increase the risk of first bleeding or even mortality.[54–56] Carvedilol is a nonselective blocker with intrinsic anti–α1-adrenergic activity that mimics the hemodynamic effects of the combination of β-blockers and prazosin.[46] Chronic carvedilol reduced HVPG by 24% and, compared with propranolol in patients without previous variceal bleeding, it increased the rate of HVPG responders from 23% to 54%.[57,58] In a randomized controlled trial, carvedilol was shown to be superior to EVL in preventing first bleeding,[59] but no face-to-face trial has compared carvedilol with β-blockers in this setting. In a proof-of-concept study, simvastatin reduced HVPG in patients with cirrhosis through a reduction in hepatic vascular resistance, an effect that adds to that of propranolol.[60] Simvastatin also has an excellent safety profile.[60]

ENDOSCOPIC THERAPY: EVL

EVL has become the endoscopic treatment of choice for the prevention of first bleeding in patients with large varices. The role of endoscopic sclerotherapy is controversial and its efficacy for primary prophylaxis is unproven despite many heterogeneous clinical trials[61] and it has been associated with a high rate of serious side effects and even greater mortality in some studies.[62] Compared with no active treatment, EVL is associated with a relative reduction in the risk of first bleeding by about 64%, and only 4 patients need to be treated with EVL to prevent a bleeding episode (see **Fig. 1**).[63,64]

Endoscopic Schedule for Variceal Eradication

There is no consensus on the most appropriate variceal eradication schedule for primary prophylaxis. Intervals between sessions vary among trials from 2 to 6 weeks. Shortening the interval between endoscopic sessions increases the risk of having to omit a session because of the presence of ulcers or nondetached bands from the previous session. In one trial, mainly including patients without previous bleeding, that compared a biweekly and bimonthly schedule of variceal eradication, a higher rate of eradication and a lower rate of recurrence were observed for the bimonthly schedule.[65] Accordingly, a recommended schedule would be monthly intervals of endoscopic sessions until eradication, and a follow-up endoscopy conducted 3 months after eradication and every 6 months thereafter.

THE CLINICAL SCENARIO OF PRIMARY PROPHYLAXIS

The Patient with Cirrhosis and Large Esophageal Varices

The most controversial issue today is whether to consider β-blockers or EVL as first-line therapy for primary prophylaxis of bleeding in patients with cirrhosis and large esophageal varices. The 2 therapies have been compared in 16 controlled trials (10 published in full[66–75] and 6 in abstract form [76–81]), with an additional trial published as a full article using carvedilol.[59] The total number of patients allocated was 1318. The studies are uniform regarding the size of varices (large varices with or without the presence of red signs), and the doses of β-blockers used. However, there were differences in variables such as sample size, length of follow-up, cause of cirrhosis, and proportion of patients with advanced liver disease. The bleeding rate was significantly lower for EVL in 5 trials,[67,71,73,79,81] whereas there were no differences between treatments in the other 11 trials using propranolol or nadolol.[66,68–70,72,74–78,80] The trial using carvedilol was the only one that showed a significant reduction in bleeding rate as a result of drug therapy.[59] Mortality was similar in both therapeutic arms in all trials, except in the trial by Jutabha and colleagues[71] in which mortality was significantly lower in the EVL group.

First bleeding was less frequent overall using EVL (EVL vs β-blockade, 13% vs 20%, and 11% vs 21% excluding the carvedilol trial). The random-effects estimate for the pooled relative risk (RR) of bleeding indicated that EVL reduced first bleeding (RR 0.64, 95% CI 0.50–0.82, and RR 0.54, 95% CI 0.41–0.71, excluding the carvedilol trial), without statistical heterogeneity (**Fig. 3**). If the analysis takes into account the time to bleeding by pooling the hazard ratio from those studies reporting time-to-event data, the favorable effect of EVL on first variceal bleeding was slightly lowered (0.64, 95% CI 0.42–0.96) or even reverted to nonsignificant when the study by Tripathi and colleagues[59] is excluded (0.84, 95% CI 0.58–1.20) (**Fig. 4**). The meta-analysis was stratified by type of publication, length of follow-up, percentage of patients with alcoholic or Child-Pugh C cirrhosis, methodological quality of trials (generation and concealment of allocation sequence, intention-to-treat analysis, description of drop-outs). In our metaregression analysis, the only covariate related to the treatment effect was concealment of the allocation sequence, with an overestimation of the effect of EVL in the 9 trials with inadequate concealment (RR 0.41, 95% CI 0.27-0.62)[66,67,73,76–81] compared with the 8 trials with adequate concealment (RR 0.88, 95% CI 0.63–1.28).[59,68–72,74,75] Pooled analysis showed a similar effect of both treatments on mortality (RR 0.97, 95% CI 0.79–1.17).

Since 2001, this issue has been the subject of several meta-analyses.[44,63,82–85] In keeping with our results, other meta-analyses have revealed a significantly lower incidences of first variceal hemorrhage in the EVL arm, without any differences in mortality.

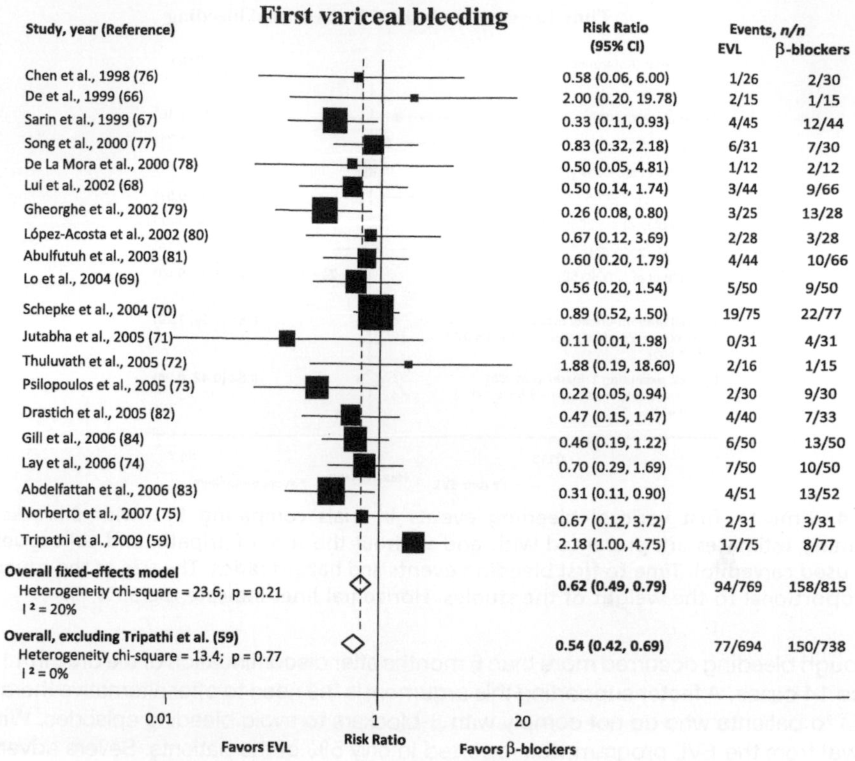

Fig. 3. First variceal bleeding events in trials comparing EVL with β-blockers. Summary estimates are presented with and without the trial of Tripathi and colleagues[59] that used carvedilol. First bleeding events and risk ratios. The size of the squares is proportional to the weight of the studies. Horizontal lines indicate the 95% CI.

These meta-analyses were stratified by type of publication (abstract or full article), quality of trial, sample size, and length of follow-up.[84,85] Summary estimates for first bleeding in these stratified meta-analyses still favored EVL when only fully published or high-quality trials were analyzed,[44,85] and were similar for the 2 treatments when only trials including more than 100 patients,[84] or with more than 20 months of follow-up, were considered.[85] However, some of the trials have been questioned for being underpowered,[84] for inadequate bias control,[85] or for early interruption (3 because of futility,[70,72,75] and 1 because of a higher rate of treatment failure in the β-blocker arm[71]).

In addition to efficacy, other aspects of therapy, such as adverse effects, cost, and quality of life, deserve consideration when evaluating treatments. Analysis of the 12 trials, those published in full,[66–75] the carvedilol trial,[59] and one of the trials published as an abstract,[80] revealed that the overall incidence of reported side effects was higher in patients on β-blockers (odds ratio 0.72, 95% CI 0.43–1.22), with significant heterogeneity detected as a result of differences in the definition, type, and severity of the adverse effects considered in each trial. β-blockers were discontinued because of side effects or intolerance in 12.3% of the patients, a percentage similar to that previously reported in trials comparing β-blockers with placebo,[43] and a similar figure (13.3%) was observed in the carvedilol trial.[59] An argument against β-blockers was the potential bleeding risk when these agents are withdrawn because of side effects or noncompliance. Fourteen of the 66 (21%) patients in whom β-blockers or carvedilol were discontinued bled,

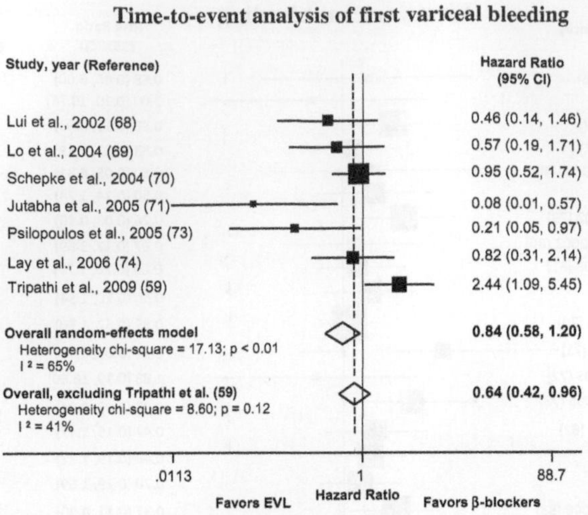

Fig. 4. Time to first variceal bleeding events in trials comparing EVL with β-blockers. Summary estimates are presented with and without the trial of Tripathi and colleagues[59] that used carvedilol. Time to first bleeding events and hazard ratios. The size of the squares is proportional to the weight of the studies. Horizontal lines indicate the 95% CI.

although bleeding occurred more than 6 months after discontinuation of the drug in 11 of these 14 cases. A factor supporting this argument is the need to offer alternative therapy (EVL) to patients who do not comply with β-blockers to avoid bleeding episodes. Withdrawal from the EVL program was reported in only 5% of the patients. Severe adverse effects (ie, requiring admission and, in most cases, also blood transfusion) were only observed at a rate of 4.9% in patients treated with EVL. These adverse effects included esophageal perforation in 1 patient, overtube laceration in 1 patient, and postbanding ulcer-related bleeding in 26 patients, and were fatal in 3 patients.[70,75] The number of side effects of EVL is probably underestimated, because the length of follow-up of most of the trials was short, and these patients needed additional endoscopies and banding sessions in the long-term. The potential harmful consequences of EVL are further indicated by the early interruption of a trial comparing EVL with no treatment in patients with contraindications to β-blockers awaiting liver transplantation because of the high incidence of postbanding ulcers.[64]

Some caveats further define what seems to be the conclusion of the meta-analyses, that EVL is more effective in preventing first bleeding than β-blockers. However, there is a potential for severe adverse effects: (1) the analyzed trials have methodological drawbacks, with a tendency to overestimate the effect of EVL in the studies of lower quality. However, at most the efficacy of both therapies is similar when low-quality trials are excluded. (2) The low sample size of the trials causes some studies to be underpowered and others prematurely interrupted. Analysis of the available evidence provides the basis for planning future research. The low number of bleeding events in cirrhotic patients with large varices on primary prophylaxis (drug or endoscopic) hinders the design of a trial of sufficient size to provide a sound response. Researchers have proposed a sample size in the range of 652 to 2000 patients.[64,84] (3) There are concerns regarding the baseline bleeding risk of the analyzed trials. The overall bleeding rate of the β-blockers arm is 20% (see **Fig. 3**), which is only slightly lower that the rate of first bleeding in untreated patients (see **Fig. 1**),[26] and this raises doubts related to the use of β-blockers in these studies. (4) The high number of patients who need to be treated to obtain a benefit with a therapy (EVL) associated with possible severe side effects. The number that need to be treated with EVL instead of β-blockers to prevent an episode of bleeding is 14 (95% CI 11–12) if we consider the trials that use propranolol or nadolol, and reaches 18 (95% CI 13–35) when the carvedilol trial is included.

Cost-effectiveness and quality of life are other factors that should be considered. EVL is an expensive procedure, requiring a mean of 3.3 sessions to achieve variceal eradication, and a surveillance endoscopy performed every 6 months to detect and ligate recurrent varices. The cost-effectiveness of β-blockers versus EVL has been evaluated in 3 decision-analysis studies, with conflicting results due to different assumptions concerning the variceal bleeding risk and quality of life related to each treatment.[23,25,86] A direct cost analysis performed in only 1 study indicated no differences between treatments[71] but was based on a small sample size and did not include the true costs incurred by the patients. A recent study examined patient preferences as an indirect measure of quality of life in patients with cirrhosis undergoing primary prophylaxis.[87] Sixty-four percent of patients and 57% of prescribing physicians preferred EVL to β-blockers. Shortness of breath or hypotension were perceived by patients and physicians as more important factors than procedure-related complications. Treatment tolerability also tended to be better for EVL throughout the follow-up in the trial by Schepke and colleagues.[70] These data reveal the importance of considering patient preferences when choosing among effective therapeutic options after discussing their benefits and risks with the patient.

Contrary to the prevention of variceal rebleeding (secondary prophylaxis),[88] the combination of β-blockers and EVL cannot be recommended for primary prophylaxis. The only trial that has compared β-blockers and EVL with EVL alone has shown that the rate of variceal recurrence is lower for combination therapy, but at the expense of a significantly increased number of side effects, and without differences in primary outcomes, bleeding, and death.[89]

In the light of the available evidence, it seems that EVL and β-blockers are effective in reducing the risk of first variceal bleeding in patients with large varices, independently of the presence of red signs. EVL seems to be more effective and is preferred by patients, but it has drawbacks including severe procedure-related complications and the need for multiple endoscopies to achieve variceal obliteration and further endoscopies during follow-up. EVL is the prophylactic therapy of choice in patients with contraindications to β-blockers. β-blockers have a more favorable safety profile and, more importantly, have a potential effect on other portal hypertension–related complications. However, noncompliance is not unusual because of drug intolerance due to systemic side effects, compromising quality of life. The decision to select EVL or β-blockers should consider patient preferences after careful explanation of the pros and cons of each therapy and physician expertise.

The Patient with Small Varices

Options in the patient with small varices include β-blockers or endoscopic surveillance without treatment (see **Table 2**). The cumulative analysis of 4 trials (454 patients) in which the effect of β-blockers in patients with small varices was addressed revealed a nonsignificant reduction in the bleeding rate in the β-blockers group compared with the placebo group (6.6% vs 10.9%, absolute risk difference 4.6%, 95% CI from −9.7% to −0.5%).[50] Differences in the definition of small varices among studies, the small sample size, and fewer bleeding events in these patients question the robustness of these data. It could also be argued that, from a cost-effectiveness perspective, early therapy with β-blockers is more beneficial than endoscopic surveillance plus treatment when varices become large. β-blockers significantly reduce growth from small to large varices.[6] In consequence, β-blockers are indicated in patients with small esophageal varices at a high risk of bleeding because of the presence of red signs or advanced liver disease (Child class C) (see **Table 2**). In other patients with small esophageal varices, a formal recommendation on the use of β-blockers cannot be made. In patients not receiving β-blockers, surveillance endoscopies should be performed every 2 years and annually if decompensation occurs, as discussed earlier.[21,43]

The Patient with Cirrhosis Without Esophageal Varices

Because increased portal pressure is the main factor promoting the appearance of esophageal varices, the hypothesis has been tested that varices formation may be avoided by lowering portal pressure in patients with cirrhosis but without varices. However, a large, multicenter, placebo-controlled, double-blinded trial failed to show a benefit of timolol (a nonselective β-blocker) in preventing variceal formation in such a population.[3] The rate of severe symptomatic adverse events was also greater in the timolol group. The trial found a reduction in the development of varices in patients showing a small (≥10% from baseline) reduction in HVPG after 1 year of treatment, and this reduction was observed in a greater proportion of patients in the timolol group. This finding suggests that there is a possibility that drugs more potent than timolol at lowering portal pressure could have an effect on variceal development. On the current evidence, β-blockers cannot be recommended for the prevention of variceal formation in patients with cirrhosis.

SUMMARY

Screening for the presence of esophageal varices is obligatory in patients with cirrhosis. Varices are common in patients with cirrhosis (30% and 60% of patients with compensated and decompensated cirrhosis, respectively) and it is associated with bleeding, if left untreated, in approximately 30% and 10% at 2 years in patients with large and small varices, respectively. Each bleeding episode is associated with a 20% mortality risk. Variceal bleeding is preventable, and identification of high-risk patients is easy with EGD. β-blockers and EVL are effective in reducing the risk of a first bleeding episode in patients with cirrhosis and large esophageal varices, and the choice in the individual patient should take into account the pros and cons of each treatment. EVL seems to be more effective in lowering the bleeding risk, but might cause severe side effects and requires endoscopic follow-up, whereas β-blockers have a better safety profile and may also reduce the risk of developing other portal hypertension–related complications. EVL is the treatment of choice in patients with contraindications or intolerance to β-blockers. β-blockers are indicated in patients with small varices with red signs or occurring in Child-Pugh class C patients, whose liver disease is classified as Child-Pugh class C, whose bleeding risk is comparable to patients with large varices. The long-term benefits of β-blockade in other patients with small varices have not been established. Prophylaxis in patients with cirrhosis without varices is not indicated, and these subjects should undergo endoscopic surveillance every 2 to 3 years. Patients in whom β-blockers reduce the HVPG to less than the threshold value have the lowest risk of first bleeding as well as a reduced risk of the other complications of portal hypertension.

REFERENCES

1. D'Amico G, Garcia-Tsao G, Pagliaro L. Natural history and prognostic indicators of survival in cirrhosis: a systematic review of 118 studies. J Hepatol 2006;44: 217–31.

2. de Franchis R. Updating consensus in portal hypertension: report of the Baveno II Consensus Workshop on definitions, methodology and therapeutic strategies in portal hypertension. J Hepatol 2000;33:846–52.
3. Groszmann RJ, García-Tsao G, Bosch J, et al. Beta-blockers to prevent gastroesophageal varices in patients with cirrhosis. N Engl J Med 2005;353: 2254–61.
4. Zoli M, Merkel C, Magalotti D, et al. Natural history of cirrhotic patients with small esophageal varices: a prospective study. Am J Gastroenterol 2000;95:503–8.
5. Merli M, Nicolini G, Angeloni S, et al. Incidence and natural history of small esophageal varices in cirrhotic patients. J Hepatol 2003;38:266–72.
6. Merkel C, Marin R, Angeli P, et al. A placebo-controlled clinical trial of nadolol in the prophylaxis of growth of small esophageal varices in cirrhosis. Gastroenterology 2004;127:476–84.
7. D'Amico G. Esophageal varices: from acceptance to rupture; natural history and prognostic indicators. In: Groszmann RJ, Bosch J, editors. Portal hypertension in the 21st century. London: Kluwer Academic Publishers; 2004. p. 147–54.
8. Carbonell N, Pauwels A, Serfaty L, et al. Improved survival after variceal bleeding in patients with cirrhosis over the past two decades. Hepatology 2004;40:652–9.
9. The North Italian Endoscopic Club for the Study and Treatment of Esophageal Varices. Prediction of the first variceal hemorrhage in patients with cirrhosis of the liver and esophageal varices. N Engl J Med 1988;31:983–9.
10. Merkel C, Zoli M, Siringo S, et al. Prognostic indicators of risk for first variceal bleeding in cirrhosis: a multicenter study in 711 patients to validate and improve the North Italian Endoscopic Club (NIEC) index. Am J Gastroenterol 2000;95: 2915–20.
11. Beppu K, Inokuchi K, Koyanagi N, et al. Prediction of variceal hemorrhage by esophageal endoscopy. Gastrointest Endosc 1981;27:213–8.
12. Idezuki Y. General rules for recording endoscopic findings of esophagogastric varices. Japanese Society for Portal Hypertension. World J Surg 1995;19: 420–2.
13. Dagradi AE, Stempien SJ, Owens LK. Bleeding esophagogastric varices. Arch Surg 1966;92:944–7.
14. Westaby D, Melia WM, MacDougal BR, et al. Injection sclerotherapy for esophageal varices. A prospective randomized trial of different treatment schedules. Gut 1984;25:129–32.
15. Winkfield B, Aubé C, Burtin P, et al. Inter-observer and intra-observer variability in hepatology. Eur J Gastroenterol Hepatol 2003;15:959–66.
16. Calès P, Oberti F, Bernard-Chabert B, et al. Evaluation of Baveno recommendations for grading esophageal varices. J Hepatol 2003;39:657–9.
17. de Franchis R, Pascal JP, Ancona E, et al. Definitions, methodology and therapeutic strategies in portal hypertension. A Consensus Development Workshop, Baveno, Lake Maggiore, Italy, April 5 and 6, 1990. J Hepatol 1992;15:256–61.
18. Madhotra R, Mulcahy HE, Willner I, et al. Prediction of esophageal varices in patients with cirrhosis. J Clin Gastroenterol 2002;34:81–5.
19. Christensen E, Fauerholdt L, Schlichting P, et al. Aspects of the natural history of gastrointestinal bleeding in cirrhosis and the effect of prednisone. Gastroenterology 1981;81:944–52.
20. D'Amico G, Garcia-Tsao G, Cales P, et al. Diagnosis of portal hypertension: how and when. In: de Franchis R. Portal hypertension III. Proceedings of the Third Baveno International Consensus Workshop on Definitions, Methodology and Therapeutic Strategies. Oxford (UK): Blackwell Science; 2001. p. 36–64.

21. García-Tsao G, Sanyal AJ, Grace ND, et al. Prevention and management of gastroesophageal varices and variceal haemorrhage in cirrhosis. AASLD Practice Guidelines. Hepatology 2007;46:922–38.
22. de Franchis R. Evolving consensus in portal hypertension. Report of the Baveno IV Consensus Workshop on methodology of diagnosis and therapy in portal hypertension. J Hepatol 2005;43:167–76.
23. Saab S, DeRosa V, Nieto J, et al. Cost and clinical outcomes of primary prophylaxis of variceal bleeding in patients with hepatic cirrhosis: a decision analytic model. Am J Gastroenterol 2003;98:763–70.
24. Spiegel BM, Targownik L, Dulai GS, et al. Endoscopic screening for esophageal varices in cirrhosis: is it ever cost effective? Hepatology 2003;37:366–77.
25. Arguedas MR, Heudebert GR, Eloubeidi MA, et al. Cost-effectiveness of screening, surveillance, and primary prophylaxis strategies for esophageal variceal bleeding. Am J Gastroenterol 2002;97:2441–52.
26. D'Amico G, Pagliaro L, Bosch J. Pharmacological treatment of portal hypertension: an evidence-based approach. Semin Liver Dis 1999;19:475–505.
27. Poynard T, Cales P, Pasta L, et al. Beta-adrenergic-antagonist drugs in the prevention of gastrointestinal bleeding in patients with cirrhosis and esophageal varices. An analysis of data and prognostic factors in 589 patients form four randomized trials. Franco-italian Multicenter study group. N Engl J Med 1991;324:1532–8.
28. Chen W, Nikolova D, Frederiksen SL, et al. Beta-blockers reduce mortality in cirrhotic patients with esophageal varices who have never bled (Cochrane review). J Hepatol 2004;40(Suppl 1):67.
29. Grozsmann RJ, García-Tsao G, Bosch J, et al. Hemodynamic events in a prospective randomized trial of propanolol versus placebo in the prevention of the first variceal hemorrhage. Gastroenterology 1990;99:1401–7.
30. Merckel C, Bolognesi M, Sacerdoti D, et al. The hemodynamic response to medical treatment of portal hypertension as a predictor of clinical effectiveness in the primary prophylaxis of variceal bleeding in cirrhosis. Hepatology 2000; 32:930–4.
31. Escorsell A, Bordas JM, Castaneda B, et al. Predictive value of the variceal pressure response to continued pharmacological therapy in patients with cirrhosis and portal hypertension. Hepatology 2000;31:1061–7.
32. Bureau C, Perón JM, Alric L, et al. "A la carte" treatment of portal hypertension of portal hypertension: adapting therapy to hemodynamic response for the prevention of bleeding. Hepatology 2002;36:1361–6.
33. Turnes J, García-Pagan JC, Abraldes JG, et al. Pharmacological reduction of portal pressure and long-term risk of first variceal bleeding in patients with cirrhosis. Am J Gastroenterol 2006;101:506–12.
34. Albillos A, Bañares R, Gonzalez M, et al. Value of hepatic venous pressure gradient to monitor drug therapy for portal hypertension: a meta-analysis. Am J Gastroenterol 2007;102:1116–26.
35. D'Amico G, Garcia-Pagan JC, Luca A, et al. Hepatic vein pressure gradient reduction and prevention of variceal bleeding in cirrhosis a systematic review. Gastroenterology 2006;131:1611–24.
36. Feu F, Garcia-Pagan JC, Bosch J, et al. Relation between portal pressure response to pharmacotherapy and risk of recurrent variceal haemorrhage in patients with cirrhosis. Lancet 1995;346:1056–9.
37. Villanueva C, Aracil C, Colomo A, et al. Acute hemodynamic response to beta-blockers and prediction of long-term outcome in primary prophylaxis of variceal bleeding. Gastroenterology 2009;137:119–28.

38. La Mura V, Abraldes JG, Raffa S, et al. Prognostic value of acute hemodynamic response to i.v. propranolol in patients with cirrhosis and portal hypertension. J Hepatol 2009;51:279–87.
39. Bosch J, Mastai R, Kravetz D, et al. Effects of propranolol on azygos venous blood flow and hepatic and systemic hemodynamics in cirrhosis. Hepatology 1984;4:1200–5.
40. Cales P, Braillon A, Jiron MI, et al. Superior portosystemic collateral circulation estimated by azygos blood flow in patients with cirrhosis. Lack of correlation with oesophageal varices and gastrointestinal bleeding. Effect of propranolol. J Hepatol 1985;1:37–46.
41. Feu F, Bordas JM, Luca A, et al. Reduction of variceal pressure by propranolol: comparison of the effects on portal pressure and azygos blood flow in patients with cirrhosis. Hepatology 1993;18:1082–9.
42. Abraczinkas DR, Ookubo R, Grace ND, et al. Propranolol for the prevention of first variceal hemorrhage: a lifetime commitment? Hepatology 2001;34: 1096–102.
43. Bolognesi M, Balducci G, Garcia-Tsao G, et al. Complications in the medical treatment of portal hypertension. Portal Hypertension III. Proceedings of the Third Baveno International Consensus Workshop on Definitions, Methodology and Therapeutic Strategies. Oxford (UK): Blackwell Science, 2001. p.180–203.
44. Khuroo MS, Khuroo NS, Farahat KL, et al. Meta-analysis: endoscopic variceal ligation for primary prophylaxis of esophageal variceal bleeding. Aliment Pharmacol Ther 2005;21:347–61.
45. García-Pagán JC, Feu F, Bosch J, et al. Propanolol compared with propanolol plus isosorbide 5-mononitrate for portal hypertension in cirrhosis. A randomized controlled study. Ann Intern Med 1991;114:869–73.
46. Albillos A, Garcia-Pagan JC, Iborra J, et al. Propranolol plus prazosin compared with propranolol plus isosorbide-5- mononitrate in the treatment of portal hypertension. Gastroenterology 1998;115:116–23.
47. Pietrosi G, D'amico G, Pasta L, et al. Isosorbide mononitrate (ISMN) with nadolol compared to nadolol alone for prevention of first variceal bleeding in cirrhosis. A double blind placebo-controlled randomized trial. J Hepatol 1999;30(S1):66.
48. Merkel C, Marin R, Sacerdoti D, et al. Long-term results of clinical trial of nadolol with or without isosorbide 5-mononitrate for primary prophylaxis of variceal bleeding in cirrhosis. Hepatology 2000;31:324–9.
49. García Pagán JC, Morillas R, Bañares R, et al. Propanolol plus placebo versus propanolol plus isosorbide 5 mononitrate in the prevention of first variceal bleed: a double blind RCT. Hepatology 2003;37:1260–6.
50. Albillos A. Pharmacological alternatives to β-blockers in primary prophylaxis. In: de Franchis R. Portal hypertension IV. Proceedings of the Fourth Baveno International Consensus Workshop on methodology of diagnosis and treatment. Oxford (UK): Blackwell; 2006. p. 177–180.
51. Abecasis R, Kravetz D, Fassio E, et al. Nadolol plus spironolactone in the prophylaxis of first variceal bleed in nonascitic cirrhotic patients: a preliminary study. Hepatology 2003;37:359–65.
52. Gonzalez-Abraldes J, Albillos A, Banares R, et al. Randomized comparison of long-term losartan versus propranolol in lowering portal pressure in cirrhosis. Gastroenterology 2001;121:382–8.
53. Schepke M, Werner E, Biecker E, et al. Hemodynamic effects of the angiotensin II receptor antagonist irbesartan in patients with cirrhosis and portal hypertension. Gastroenterology 2001;121:389–95.

54. Angelico M, Carli L, Piat C, et al. Effects of isosorbide-5-mononitrate compared with propranolol on first bleeding and long-term survival in cirrhosis. Gastroenterology 1997;113:1632–9.
55. Garcia-Pagan JC, Villanueva C, Vila MC, et al. Isosorbide mononitrate in the prevention of first variceal bleed in patients who cannot receive beta-blockers. Gastroenterology 2001;121:908–14.
56. Borroni G, Salerno F, Cazzaniga M, et al. Nadolol is superior to isosorbide mononitrate for the prevention of the first variceal bleeding in cirrhotic patients with ascites. J Hepatol 2002;37:315–21.
57. Bañares R, Moitinho E, Piqueras B, et al. Carvedilol, a new nonselective beta-blocker with intrinsic anti-Alpha1-adrenergic activity, has a greater portal hypotensive effect than propranolol in patients with cirrhosis. Hepatology 1999;30: 79–83.
58. Tripathi D, Therapondos G, Lui HF, et al. Haemodynamic effects of acute and chronic administration of low-dose carvedilol, a vasodilating beta-blocker, in patients with cirrhosis and portal hypertension. Aliment Pharmacol Ther 2002; 16:373–80.
59. Tripathi D, Ferguson JW, Kochar N, et al. Randomized controlled trial of carvedilol versus variceal band ligation for the prevention of the first variceal bleed. Hepatology 2009;50:825–33.
60. Abraldes JG, Albillos A, Bañares R, et al. Simvastatin lowers portal pressure in patients with cirrhosis and portal hypertension: a randomized controlled trial. Gastroenterology 2009;136:1651–8.
61. Pagliaro L, D'Amico G, Sörensen TI, et al. Prophylaxis of first bleeding. A meta-analysis of randomized trials of nonsurgical treatment. Ann Intern Med 1992; 117:59–70.
62. The Veterans Affairs Cooperative Variceal Sclerotherapy Group. Prophylactic sclerotherapy for esophageal varices in men with alcoholic liver disease. A randomized, single-blind, multicenter clinical trial. N Engl J Med 1991;324: 1779–84.
63. Imperiale TF, Chalasani N. A meta-analysis of endoscopic variceal ligation for primary prophylaxis of esophageal variceal bleeding. Hepatology 2001;33: 802–7.
64. Triantos C, Vlachogiannakos J, Armonis A, et al. Primary prophylaxis of variceal bleeding in cirrhotics unable to take β-blockers: a randomized trial of ligation. Aliment Pharmacol Ther 2005;21:1435–43.
65. Yoshida H, Mamada Y, Taniai N, et al. A randomized control trial of bi-monthly versus bi-weekly endoscopic variceal ligation of esophageal varices. Am J Gastroenterol 2005;100:2005–9.
66. De BK, Ghoshal UC, Das T, et al. Endoscopic variceal ligation for primary prophylaxis of esophageal variceal bleed: preliminary report of a randomized controlled trial. J Gastroenterol Hepatol 1999;14:220–4.
67. Sarin SK, Lamba GS, Kumar M, et al. Comparison of endoscopic ligation and propanolol for the primary prevention of variceal bleeding. N Engl J Med 1999; 340:988–93.
68. Lui HF, Stanley AJ, Forrest EH, et al. Primary prophylaxis of variceal hemorrhage: a randomized controlled trial comparing band ligation, propanolol and isosorbide mononitrate. Gastroenterology 2002;123:735–44.
69. Lo GH, Chen W, Chen MH, et al. Endoscopic ligation vs. nadolol in the prevention of first variceal bleeding in patients with cirrhosis. Gastrointest Endosc 2004;59: 333–8.

70. Schepke M, Kleber G, Nurnberg D, et al. Ligation vs. propanolol for the primary prophylaxis of variceal bleeding in cirrhosis. Hepatology 2004;40:65–72.
71. Jutabha R, Jensen DM, Martin P, et al. Randomized study comparing banding and propanolol to prevent initial variceal haemorrhage in cirrhotics with high-risk esophageal varices. Gastroenterology 2005;128:870–81.
72. Thuluvath PJ, Maheshwari A, Jagannath S, et al. A randomized controlled trial of beta-blockers versus endoscopic band ligation for primary prophylaxis: a large sample size is required to show difference in bleeding rates. Dig Dis Sci 2005; 50:407–10.
73. Psilopoulos D, Galanis P, Goulas S, et al. Endoscopic variceal ligation for prevention of first variceal bleeding: a randomized controlled trial. Eur J Gastroenterol Hepatol 2005;17:1111–7.
74. Lay CS, Tsai YT, Lee FY, et al. Endoscopic variceal ligation versus propanolol in prophylaxis of first variceal bleeding in patients with cirrhosis. J Gastroenterol Hepatol 2006;21:413–9.
75. Norberto L, Polese L, Cillo U, et al. A randomized study comparing ligation with propanolol for primary prophylaxis of variceal bleeding in candidates for liver transplantation. Liver Transpl 2007;13:1272–8.
76. Chen C, Sheu M, Su S. Prophylactic endoscopic variceal ligation (EVL) with multiple band ligator for esophageal varices. Gastroenterology 1998;144: A1224.
77. Song I, Shin J, Kim I, et al. A prospective randomized trial between the prophylactic endoscopic variceal ligation and propanolol administration for prevention of first bleeding in cirrhotic patients with high-risk esophageal varices. J Hepatol 2000;32(Suppl 2):41.
78. De la Mora J, Farca-Belsaguy A, Uribe M, et al. Ligation vs. propanolol for primary prophylaxis of variceal bleeding using a multiple band ligator and objective measurements of treatment adequacy: preliminary results. Gastroenterology 2000;118:6512A.
79. Gheorge C, Gheorge L, Vadan R, et al. Prophylactic banding ligation of high risk esophageal varices in patients on the waiting list for liver transplantation: an interim report. J Hepatol 2002;36(Suppl 1):38.
80. Drastich P, Lata J, Petryl J, et al. Endoscopic variceal band ligation in comparison with propanolol in prophylaxis of first variceal bleeding in patients with liver cirrhosis. J Hepatol 2005;42(Suppl 2):79.
81. Abdelfattah MH, Rashed MA, Elfakhry AA, et al. Endoscopic variceal ligation versus pharmacological treatment for primary prophylaxis of variceal bleeding: a randomized study. J Hepatol 2006;44(Suppl 2):83A.
82. García-Pagán JC, Bosch J. Endoscopic band ligation in the treatment of portal hypertension. Nature Clin Pract Gastroenterol Hepatol 2005;2:526–35.
83. Albillos A. Preventing first variceal hemorrhage in cirrhosis. J Clin Gastroenterol 2007;41(Suppl 3):S305–311.
84. Bosch J, Berzigotti A, García-Pagán JC, et al. The management of portal hypertension: rational basis, available treatments and future options. J Hepatol 2008; 48(Suppl):S68–92.
85. Gluud LL, Klingenberg S, Nikolova D, et al. Banding ligation versus beta-blockers as primary prophylaxis in esophageal varices: systemic review of randomized trials. Am J Gastroenterol 2007;102:2841–9.
86. Imperiale TF, Klein RW, Chalasani N. Cost-effectiveness analysis of variceal ligation vs. Beta-blockers for primary prevention of variceal bleeding in patients with cirrhosis. Hepatology 2007;45:870–8.

87. Longacre AV, Imaeda A, Garcia-Tsao G, et al. A pilot project examining the predicted preferences of patients and physicians in the primary prophylaxis of variceal hemorrhage. Hepatology 2008;47:169–76.
88. González R, Zamora J, Gomez-Camarero J, et al. Meta-analysis: combination endoscopic and drug therapy to prevent variceal rebleeding in cirrhosis. Ann Intern Med 2008;149:109–22.
89. Sarin SK, Wadhawan M, Agarwal SR, et al. Endoscopic variceal ligation plus propranolol versus endoscopic variceal ligation alone in primary prophylaxis of variceal bleeding. Am J Gastroenterol 2005;100:797–804.

Management of Acute Variceal Bleeding: Emphasis on Endoscopic Therapy

Andrés Cárdenas, MD, MMSc

KEYWORDS

- Acute variceal bleeding • Endoscopic therapy
- Endoscopy • Portal hypertension • Endoscopic band ligation
- Endoscopic sclerotherapy • Cirrhosis

An abnormal increase of portal venous pressure, which may occur in subjects with or without cirrhosis, defines what is termed as portal hypertension. In portal hypertension the gradient between portal pressure and inferior vena cava pressure, the hepatic venous pressure gradient (HVPG), is increased over the normal value of 5 mm Hg. Clinically significant portal hypertension occurs when manifestations of the disease appear or when the HVPG exceeds a threshold value of 10 mm Hg.[1] Portal hypertension may occur at either prehepatic, intrahepatic, or posthepatic sites. Cirrhosis as an intrahepatic cause accounts for nearly 90% of cases. The development of portal hypertension in cirrhosis marks a milestone in the natural course of the disease as its consequences range from the development of gastroesophageal varices, variceal bleeding, ascites, hepatorenal syndrome, and hepatic encephalopathy. Variceal bleeding usually occurs late in the natural history of portal hypertension. The initial appearance of varices in patients with compensated cirrhosis indicates a progression of the disease from a low-risk state to an intermediate one. Once bleeding occurs, this indicates decompensation and progression to a high risk of death.[2] Although mortality rates from an episode of variceal bleeding have dropped from 60% to 20% at 6 weeks in the past 3 decades, an episode of acute variceal bleeding (AVB) may be associated with recurrence and other complications of end-stage liver disease.[3,4] In this context, endoscopy plays a key role in the management of AVB. Current available methods allow control of bleeding in 85% to 90% of cases within the first days of the index bleed.[5] Still, there is a risk of rebleeding within the first 6 weeks. Late rebleeding occurs in about 60% of

GI Unit / Institut Clinic de Malalties Digestives i Metaboliques, University of Barcelona, Hospital Clinic, Villarroel 170, Barcelona 08036, Spain
E-mail address: acardena@clinic.ub.es

Clin Liver Dis 14 (2010) 251–262
doi:10.1016/j.cld.2010.03.002

untreated patients within 1 to 2 years, and death occurs in nearly 30%.[6] Consequently, all patients surviving an AVB should receive secondary prophylaxis, see the article by Dr Lo elsewhere in this issue for further exploration of this topic. This article reviews current management approach of patients with AVB with particular emphasis on endoscopic treatments for bleeding varices.

NATURAL HISTORY AND DIAGNOSIS

Variceal bleeding is the final consequence of a series of steps that begin with an increase in portal pressure with the initial appearance of small varices and then their progressive dilation (at a rate of 5% per year) until they rupture.[7] Esophageal varices are present in nearly 30% to 40% of patients with compensated cirrhosis and in 60% of those with decompensated cirrhosis.[8] Patients with varices have an incidence of AVB that ranges from 4% to 15% per year depending on the severity of liver disease, variceal size, presence of red wale marks, and an HVPG value greater than 12 mm Hg.[8–10]

Patients with cirrhosis who present with an episode of upper gastrointestinal bleeding will have varices as the culprit in 70% to 80% of cases.[11] Therefore, upper gastrointestinal bleeding in a cirrhotic patient must be presumed to be variceal until proven otherwise. The gold standard for diagnosis is upper endoscopy, which may show one of the following[1]: active blood spurting or oozing from a varix, which is present in nearly 20% of patients (**Fig. 1**); white nipple or clot adherent to a varix; or presence of varices without other potential sources of bleeding in the stomach or duodenum. Although acute bleeding from varices may cease spontaneously in nearly half of patients, rebleeding rates are significantly high (30%–40%) if patients are not treated.[6,12,13] The highest risk occurs within the first 2 to 3 days after the index bleed and most of the rebleeding episodes occur within the first 14 days. After 6 weeks, the risk of further bleeding is similar to that before the index bleed.[1,13] Initial failure to control bleeding (5-day control) occurs more commonly in patients with Child class C cirrhosis, bacterial infection, portal vein thrombosis, active spurting of a varix, and an HVPG greater than 20 mm Hg.[11,14–17] Mortality rates from AVB have dropped dramatically in the past 3 decades from 42% in the 1980s[13] to the current rates of 15% to 20%,[3,4,18,19] likely because of improvements in intensive care, pharmacologic and endoscopic therapy, implementation of transjugular intrahepatic portosystemic shunts (TIPS), and prophylaxis for bacterial infections. Current estimates of mortality

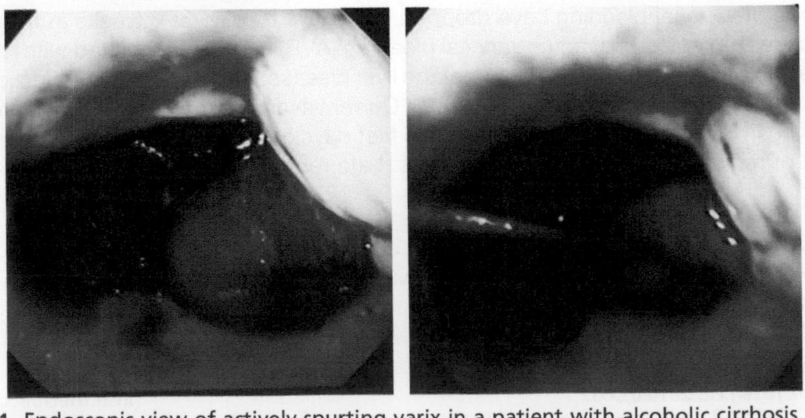

Fig. 1. Endoscopic view of actively spurting varix in a patient with alcoholic cirrhosis.

from uncontrolled bleeding are 4% to 8%.[11] Approximately one-third of deaths are a direct consequence of bleeding and the remaining are caused by liver failure, infections, and renal failure.[11,20]

Recent studies stress the importance of prognostic markers in patients with an episode of acute bleeding. The presence of an HVPG greater than 20 mm Hg, systolic blood pressure at admission lower than 100 mm Hg, and nonalcoholic cause of cirrhosis are associated with 5-day failure to control bleeding.[16] Nonetheless, clinical variables (without HVPG) associated with 5-day failure to control bleeding are advanced Child-Pugh class, systolic blood pressure of lower than 100 mm Hg on admission, and nonalcoholic etiology of cirrhosis. Both of these models have a good and very similar discriminative ability.[16] This means that upon admission, the presence of those variables will help plan ahead aggressive management and further therapies that may be needed if there is no good response to initial standard of care treatment.

GENERAL MANAGEMENT

Critical steps in the management of patients with AVB reside in providing hemodynamic resuscitation with correction of hypovolemia, preventing complications and stopping the hemorrhage. They need to be coordinated simultaneously by a multispecialty team including a hepatologist/gastroenterologist, endoscopist, critical care specialist, surgeon, and an interventional radiologist. An integrated approach that involves adequate volume resuscitation, possible endotracheal intubation, prophylactic antibiotics, administration of vasoconstrictors, and therapeutic endoscopy must be set in place by the team caring for the patient.

Resuscitation needs to be provided by the *airway, breathing, circulation* algorithm. In all cases the airway needs to be carefully evaluated and a decision of securing the airway should be made early on, especially in patients with changes in mental status, encephalopathy, and actively vomiting blood because of the high risk of aspiration. Tracheal intubation is mandatory if there is any concern about the safety of the airway.[21,22]

Volume resuscitation with plasma expanders should be instituted to keep systolic blood pressure at 100 mm Hg.[23] Avoidance of shock prevents renal failure, which is associated with an increased risk of death.[20] On the other hand, overtransfusion should be avoided because it theoretically may induce rebound increases in portal pressure and rebleeding.[23,24] Blood transfusions should aim for a hemoglobin level of 7 to 8 g/L, except in patients with active ongoing bleeding or with ischemic heart disease.[23] There are no data to support the routine use of platelet transfusion or fresh frozen plasma administration and they should be evaluated on a case-by-case basis. In patients with a platelet count lower than 50,000 per μL or with an international normalized ratio (INR) greater than 1.5, it is prudent to consider transfusion of platelets and/or plasma before the procedure weighing in the risks and benefits. Bacterial infections are a poor prognostic indicator in acute variceal bleeding.[14] The most common infections are spontaneous bacterial peritonitis, urinary tract infections, and pneumonia. Prophylactic antibiotics in patients with AVB have been shown to reduce the risk of rebleeding and mortality[25–27]; therefore, all patients on admission should receive them. Norfloxacin 400 mg orally twice daily for 7 days may be given; however, patients with hypovolemic shock, ascites, malnutrition, encephalopathy, or bilirubin greater than 3 mg/dL should receive intravenous ceftriaxone (1 g per day), as it is more effective than oral norfloxacin in the prophylaxis of bacterial infections in patients with advanced cirrhosis and AVB.[27]

Prompt initiation of vasoactive drugs (see the following section) and timing of endoscopy should be planned soon after hospitalization. Emergency endoscopy should be performed within the first 12 hours of admission.[23] If patients are actively vomiting blood, endoscopy should be performed as soon as possible once the patient has been stabilized in a monitored unit.

SPECIFIC TREATMENT

Vasocontrictors

In suspected variceal bleeding, vasoactive drugs need to be given as soon as possible and before endoscopy. This is supported by randomized controlled trials demonstrating that the early use of vasoactive drugs reduces the rate of active bleeding, making endoscopy easier to perform for diagnostic and therapeutic purposes.[28–31] Vasoactive drugs are administered because of their ability to reduce portal pressure and decrease variceal blood flow. Two types of drugs are used: vasopressin and its analogs (terlipressin) and somatostatin and its analogs (octreotide/vapreotide) (**Table 1**). Intravenous vasopressin causes vasoconstriction and decreases portal pressures. When administered with percutaneous nitroglycerin it may help achieve initial hemostasis in 70% of patients. Unfortunately it has minimal effects on early rebleeding episodes, does not improve survival, and has important ischemic side effects that limit its use. Terlipressin is a synthetic analog of vasopressin with a better safety profile. It is a selective vasoconstrictor of the splanchnic circulation that is slowly released into the circulation. Intravenous terlipressin is the preferred choice, as it is the only therapy that improves survival.[28,29] The recommend dose is 2 mg every 4 hours for the first 2 days and may be reduced afterwards to 1 mg every 4 hours for up to 5 days.[31] Side effects may include transient abdominal pain as well as self-limited diarrhea. Serious side effects such as myocardial ischemia are rare. The overall efficacy of terlipressin in controlling acute variceal bleeding at 48 hours is about 80%.[29]

Somatostatin inhibits the release of glucagon, a vasodilator hormone, which leads to splanchnic vasoconstriction and decreased portal inflow. Intravenous somatostatin is given as an initial bolus of 250 μg followed by a 250-μg per hour infusion that may be continued for up to 5 days to prevent early rebleeding.[30,32] Some side effects such as nausea, vomiting, and hyperglycemia may occur in up to one-third of patients.[30,32,33] Although it improves control of bleeding, it does not reduce mortality from AVB compared with placebo or other nonpharmacologic treatments.[12,30] Octreotide, a commonly used somatostatin analog in the United States, has a longer half-life than somatostatin.[34] The recommended doses are an initial bolus of 50 to 100 μg,

Table 1
Vasoconstrictors used in acute variceal bleeding

Drug	Dose
Vasopressin and nitroglycerin	Vasopressin IV infusion at 0.4 units/min Percutaneous nitroglycerin 20 mg
Terlipressin	IV bolus 2 mg/4 h for 24–48 h, then 1 mg/4 h
Somatostatin	IV bolus 250 μg followed by infusion of 250–500 μg/h
Octreotide	IV bolus of 50–100 μg followed by infusion of 50 μg/h
Vapreotide	IV bolus of 50 μg followed by infusion of 50 μg/h

All drugs are administered for a minimum of 2 days and may be prolonged for up to 5 days.
Abbreviation: IV, intravenous.

followed by an infusion of 50 μg per hour that can be maintained for up to 5 days. Octreotide is safe and few major side effects are reported. A limitation of octreotide is that data from meta-analyses are inconclusive and controversial.[30,34] Tachyphylaxis is another limitation.[35] When combined with endoscopic sclerotherapy, octreotide has a beneficial and significant effect in reducing early rebleeding.[34]

Endoscopy

Endoscopy is one of the cornerstones of management as it confirms the diagnosis and allows therapy during the same session. Endoscopic therapies for varices aim to reduce variceal wall tension by obliteration of the varix. The 2 endoscopic methods available for AVB are endoscopic sclerotherapy (ES) and band ligation (EBL) (**Fig. 2**).

Endoscopic sclerotherapy

ES consists of the injection of a sclerosing agent into the variceal lumen (intravariceal) or adjacent to it (paravariceal) using a freehand technique (see **Fig. 2**). This causes thrombosis of the varix and inflammation of the surrounding mucosa that creates a scar over the esophageal wall. ES is relatively easy to perform; only a flexible catheter with a short needle tip (23 or 25 gauge) and the sclerosant solution are needed. A variety of sclerosant solutions may be used. The most common are ethanolamine oleate (5%) or polidocanol (1%–2%) in Europe, and sodium morrhuate (5%) in the United States.[36,37] The first injection of 1 to 2 mL of the sclerosant should be placed right below the bleeding site. Afterward, 1- to 2-mL injections of the remaining varices adjacent to the bleeding varix are performed. The main objective is to target the lower esophagus near the gastroesophageal (GE) junction. Up to 10 to 15 mL of a sclerosant solution may be used in the session. In the acute setting, the paravariceal injection technique cannot be easily performed because of the ongoing bleeding and it is mostly reserved for elective sclerotherapy.

The advantages of ES are that is it easy to use, the injection catheter fits through the working channel of a diagnostic gastroscope, it can be quickly assembled, and does not require a second oral intubation. Additionally, there is rapid formation of

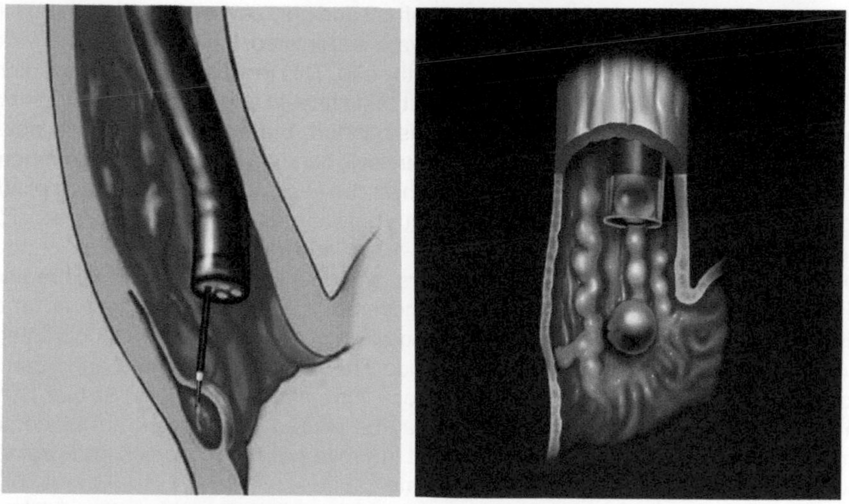

Fig. 2. Endoscopic techniques for treating esophageal varices. Endoscopic sclerotherapy (*right*) and endoscopic band ligation (*left*). (*Courtesy of* AGA GastroSlides, with permission. Copyright © AGA Institute, all rights reserved.)

a thrombus. Disadvantages include a variety of local and systemic complications. Immediate problems include substernal chest pain, fever, dysphagia, and pleural effusion.[38] Esophageal ulcers are common and in 20% of patients they may cause bleeding.[38,39] Bacteremia may occur in up to 35% and lead to other complications such as spontaneous bacterial peritonitis or distal abscesses.[40,41] Other complications include esophageal strictures, perforations, mediastinitis, pericarditis, chylothorax, esophageal motility disorders, and acute respiratory distress syndrome.[36–39]

Endoscopic band ligation

EBL was developed as an alternative, with fewer complications than ES, for the treatment of esophageal varices. It consists of the placement of elastic bands on the varices to occlude the varix and cause thrombosis.[42,43] This causes necrosis of the mucosa and the bands eventually fall off in a few days leaving a superficial mucosal ulceration that heals and eventually scars.[44] Repeat sessions are performed at 2- to 4-week intervals to reduce the risk of rebleeding, see the article by Dr Lo elsewhere in this issue for further exploration of this topic. Clinical trials of EBL demonstrate fewer side effects than ES in the treatment of esophageal varices.[45] Interestingly, HVPG transiently falls after EBL, whereas it increases with ES.[46]

Several commercial multiband devices are available for EBL; the most common are the Saeed Multiple Ligator (Wilson-Cook Medical, Inc, Winston-Salem, NC, USA) and the Speedband (Microvasive Boston Scientific Corporation, Natick, MA, USA). They have between 4 and 10 preloaded bands. All have the same principle; that is, placement of elastic bands on a varix after it is sucked into a clear plastic cylinder attached to the tip of the endoscope. Patients should receive intravenous sedation with either a benzodiazepine (midazolam) plus an opiate (meperidine or fentanyl) or propofol see the article by Dr Cohen elsewhere in this issue for further exploration of this topic. After the diagnostic endoscopy is performed and the culprit varix identified and its distance measured to the mouth, the endoscope is withdrawn and the ligation device is loaded. The device is firmly attached to the scope and placed in a neutral mode. Sometimes passing the endoscope with the loading device may be tricky. This requires slight flexion of the neck, gentle and constant advancement of the scope with visualization of the pharynx, and a slight torque of the shaft left and right. After intubation, the device is placed in "forward only" mode. Once the varix is identified, the tip is pointed toward it and continuous suction applied so it can fill the cap. This requires smooth movements right and left. Once inside the cap, a "red out" sign should appear and at this point the band can be fired (**Fig. 3**). After the varix is banded, the endoscope should not be advanced farther to avoid dislodgement. Therefore, banding should always commence in the most distal portion of the esophagus near the GE junction. Bands are applied in a spiral pattern progressing up the esophagus until all major columns of varices of the lower third of the esophagus (no more than 8–10 cm above the GE junction) are banded.

During an acute episode (see **Fig. 1**) there may be a limited view and this requires active flushing with water and suction as necessary. A band should be fired at the actively bleeding site but if missed, banding of mucosa is not harmful in contrast to injecting a sclerosant, which may cause side effects. In most cases bands can be placed at the GE junction, which may reduce torrential bleeding and further bands can be fired afterward. Up to 10 bands may be placed in 1 session but placement of more than 6 bands per session does not improve patient outcomes and prolongs procedure time and increases the misfire rate.[47]

Complications of EBL include transient dysphagia and chest pain, which are common and respond well to liquid analgesics (acetaminophen) as well as an oral suspension of antacids. Patients should start with liquids for the first 12 hours and

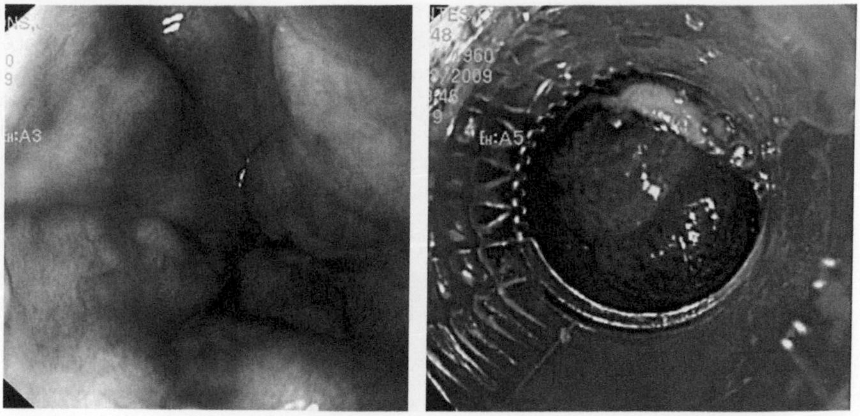

Fig. 3. Endoscopic view of large varices with red spots (*left*) and endoscopic view of a successfully placed band in a varix (*right*).

then progress with soft foods. Shallow ulcers at the site of bands are frequent but rarely bleed. The use of a proton pump inhibitor (ie, pantoprazole 40 mg per day for 10 days) decreases the size of ulcers but does not prevent them from bleeding.[48] Severe and rare complications such as massive bleeding from ulcers or rarely from variceal rupture, esophageal perforation, esophageal strictures, or altered esophageal motility, may occur with EBL.[49]

Combination therapy

A meta-analysis of 15 trials comparing emergency EST and vasoconstrictor drugs with more than 500 patients in each arm, showed a similar efficacy with both treatments, and fewer side effects with pharmacologic therapy.[50] Nonetheless, combination of both pharmacologic and endoscopic therapy in the treatment of AVB is strongly supported by numerous trials showing that the efficacy of both emergency EST and EBL is significantly improved when they are associated with pharmacologic treatment.[5,12] Although both methods are highly effective in controlling AVB, EBL has become the treatment of choice both for controlling variceal hemorrhage and for variceal obliteration in secondary prophylaxis.[5,23,51] A meta-analysis has shown that EBL is better than EST for all major outcomes including initial control of bleeding, recurrent bleeding, side effects, time to variceal obliteration, and survival.[45] Thus, combination therapy with a vasoactive drug plus EBL is considered the standard of care for AVB and it is currently recommended by guidelines.[23,51] Combination therapy improves the 5-day success rate compared with endoscopic ligation therapy alone,[52,53] but this is not associated with any differences in mortality. Given these reasons, EBL at present is the endoscopic method of choice to treat esophageal varices in most cases. However, ES is an accepted method if EBL cannot be performed.

Other Methods

Balloon tamponade of the esophagus may be required in patients with uncontrollable bleeding or those patients with such massive and profuse bleeding in whom an upper endoscopy cannot be performed. Pneumatic compression of the fundus and the lower esophagus stops bleeding in approximately 85% of cases. The problem is that recurrence after its deflation, which has to occur within 48 hours of placement, is high and major complications including aspiration pneumonia and esophageal perforation may

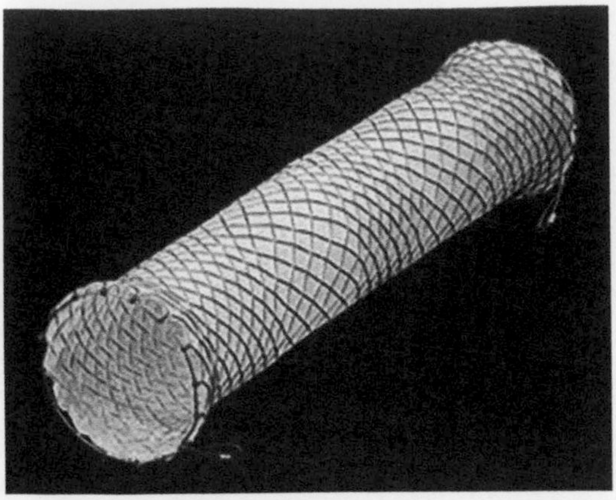

Fig. 4. A fully covered self-expandable esophageal stent can be placed in the esophagus as a rescue therapy in patients in whom variceal bleeding cannot be controlled with endoscopic band ligation or endoscopic sclerotherapy.

occur in up to 20% to 30% of patients.[54] Given the high success of current endoscopic and pharmacologic therapies, balloon tamponade is now rarely used. The recent introduction of a fully covered self-expandable metallic stent (Ella-Danis, Hradec Kralove, Czech Republic) for AVB may be useful in those cases where balloon tamponade is considered (**Fig. 4**).[55] The stent is placed over a guide wire previously passed to the stomach. The stent has a distal balloon that inflated with a syringe to ensure proper location in the cardias and lower esophagus so no fluoroscopy is needed. The stent can be left in place for up to 14 days and it can be retrieved by endoscopy with a hook system. There are limited data with its use. A pilot study of 20 patients who failed standard of care treatment reported 100% success without any significant complications. Although promising, more data are needed to consider this stent in the therapeutic armamentarium for AVB.

Failures

Approximately 10% to 15% of patients do not respond to the current first-line therapies. In such cases if the patient is stable, a second therapeutic endoscopy may be performed. However, if this is unsuccessful or there is massive bleeding, the patient

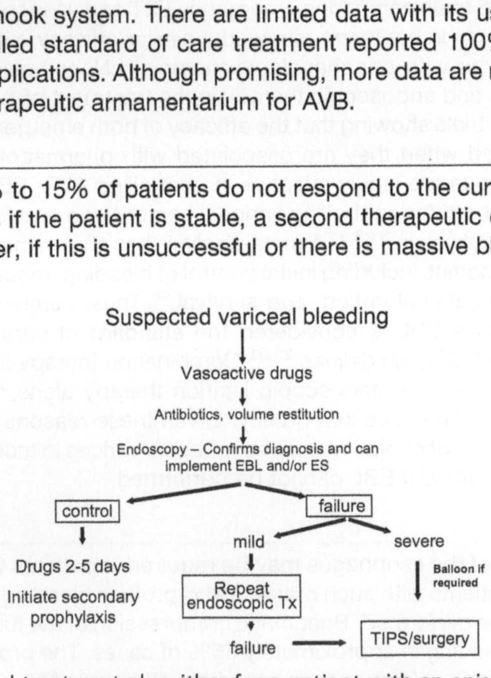

Fig. 5. Recommended treatment algorithm for a patient with an episode of acute variceal bleeding.

should be considered for other treatments. This topic is discussed in detail, see the article by Dr Garcia-Pagan and colleagues elsewhere in this issue for further exploration of this topic.

SUMMARY

AVB is a dreaded complication of patients with portal hypertension. Initial management includes appropriate volume replacement, transfusion of blood to keep hemoglobin levels at 8 g/L, antibiotic prophylaxis, and endotracheal intubation in selected cases. Standard of care mandates for early administration of vasoactive drug therapy and then EBL or injection ES (if EBL cannot be performed) within the first 12 hours of the index bleed. The use of pharmacologic agents may be prolonged for up to 5 days. Patients who fail endoscopic therapy may require temporary placement of balloon tamponade; however, its use is associated with potentially lethal complications such as aspiration and perforation of the esophagus. Therefore, it should be placed in experienced units and should be followed by a more definitive therapy. All patients surviving an episode of AVB should undergo further prophylaxis to prevent rebleeding. The current management of AVB is summarized in **Fig. 5.**

REFERENCES

1. Bosch J, Garcia-Pagan JC, Berzigotti A, et al. Measurement of portal pressure and its role in the management of chronic liver disease. Semin Liver Dis 2006; 26:348–62.
2. D'Amico G, Garcia-Tsao G, Pagliaro L. Natural history and prognostic indicators of survival in cirrhosis: a systematic review of 118 studies. J Hepatol 2006;44: 217–31.
3. Chalasani N, Kahi C, Francois F, et al. Improved patient survival after acute variceal bleeding: a multicenter, cohort study. Am J Gastroenterol 2003;98:653–9.
4. Carbonell N, Pauwels A, Serfaty L, et al. Improved survival after variceal bleeding in patients with cirrhosis over the past two decades. Hepatology 2004;40:652–9.
5. Qureshi W, Adler DG, Davila R, et al. ASGE guideline: the role of endoscopy in the management of variceal hemorrhage, updated. Gastrointest Endosc 2005; 2005(62):651–5.
6. Bosch J, Garcia-Pagan JC. Prevention of variceal rebleeding. Lancet 2003;361: 952–4.
7. Merli M, Nicolini G, Angeloni S, et al. Incidence and natural history of small esophageal varices in cirrhotic patients. J Hepatol 2003;38:266–72.
8. de Franchis R, Primignani M. Natural history of portal hypertension in patients with cirrhosis. Clin Liver Dis 2001;5(3):645–63.
9. The North Italian Endoscopic Club for the Study and Treatment of Esophageal Varices. Prediction of the first variceal hemorrhage in patients with cirrhosis of the liver and esophageal varices. A prospective multicenter study. N Engl J Med 1988;319:983–9.
10. Groszmann RJ, Bosch J, Grace ND, et al. Hemodynamic events in a prospective randomized trial of propranolol versus placebo in the prevention of a first variceal hemorrhage. Gastroenterology 1990;99:1401–7.
11. D'Amico G, de Franchis R. Upper digestive bleeding in cirrhosis. Post-therapeutic outcome and prognostic indicators. Hepatology 2003;38:599–612.
12. D'Amico G, Pagliaro L, Bosch J. Pharmacological treatment of portal hypertension: an evidence-based approach. Semin Liver Dis 1999;19:475–505.

13. Graham D, Smith J. The course of patients after variceal hemorrhage. Gastroenterology 1981;80:800–6.
14. Goulis J, Armonis A, Patch D, et al. Bacterial infection is independently associated with failure to control bleeding in cirrhotic patients with gastrointestinal hemorrhage. Hepatology 1998;27:1207–12.
15. Ben Ari Z, Cardin F, McCormick AP, et al. A predictive model for failure to control bleeding during acute variceal haemorrhage. J Hepatol 1999;31:443–50.
16. Abraldes JG, Villanueva C, Banares R, et al. Hepatic venous pressure gradient and prognosis in patients with acute variceal bleeding treated with pharmacologic and endoscopic therapy. J Hepatol 2008;48:229–36.
17. Monescillo A, Martinez-Lagares F, Ruiz-del-Arbol L. Influence of portal hypertension and its early decompression by TIPS placement on the outcome of variceal bleeding. Hepatology 2004;40:793–801.
18. Stokkeland K, Brandt L, Ekbom A, et al. Improved prognosis for patients hospitalized with esophageal varices in Sweden 1969–2002. Hepatology 2006;43:500–5.
19. Bambha K, Kim WR, Pedersen R, et al. Predictors of early re-bleeding and mortality after acute variceal haemorrhage in patients with cirrhosis. Gut 2008; 57:814–20.
20. Cardenas A, Gines P, Uriz J, et al. Renal failure after upper gastrointestinal bleeding in cirrhosis: incidence, clinical course, predictive factors, and short-term prognosis. Hepatology 2001;34:671–6.
21. Koch DG, Arguedas MR, Fallon MB. Risk of aspiration pneumonia in suspected variceal hemorrhage: the value of prophylactic endotracheal intubation prior to endoscopy. Dig Dis Sci 2007;52:2225–8.
22. Rudolph SJ, Landsverk BK, Freeman ML. Endotracheal intubation for airway protection during endoscopy for severe upper GI hemorrhage. Gastrointest Endosc 2003;57:58–61.
23. de Franchis R. Evolving consensus in portal hypertension: report of the Baveno IV consensus workshop on methodology of diagnosis and therapy in portal hypertension. J Hepatol 2005;43:167–76.
24. Castaneda B, Debernardi-Venon W, Bandi JC. The role of portal pressure in the severity of bleeding in portal hypertensive rats. Hepatology 2000;31:581–6.
25. Hou MC, Lin HC, Liu TT. Antibiotic prophylaxis after endoscopic therapy prevents rebleeding in acute variceal hemorrhage: a randomized trial. Hepatology 2004; 39:746–53.
26. Soares-Weiser K, Brezis M, Tur-Kaspa R, et al. Antibiotic prophylaxis of bacterial infections in cirrhotic inpatients: a meta-analysis of randomized controlled trials. Scand J Gastroenterol 2003;38(2):193–200.
27. Fernandez J, Ruiz-del-Arbol L, Gomez C, et al. Norfloxacin vs ceftriaxone in the prophylaxis of infections in patients with advanced cirrhosis and hemorrhage. Gastroenterology 2006;131:1049–56.
28. Levacher S, Letoumelin P, Pateron D, et al. Early administration of terlipressin plus glyceryl trinitrate to control active upper gastrointestinal bleeding in cirrhotic patients. Lancet 1995;346:865–8.
29. Ioannou G, Doust J, Rockey DC. Terlipressin for acute variceal hemorrhage. Cochrane Database Syst Rev 2003;1:CD002147.
30. Gotzsche PC, Hrobjartsson A. Somatostatin analogues for acute bleeding oesophageal varices. Cochrane Database Syst Rev 2008;3:CD000193.
31. Escorsell A, Ruiz-del-Arbol L, Planas R, et al. Multicenter randomized controlled trial of terlipressin versus sclerotherapy in the treatment of acute variceal bleeding: the TEST study. Hepatology 2000;32:471–6.

32. Escorsell A, Bordas JM, del Arbol LR, et al. Randomized controlled trial of sclerotherapy versus somatostatin infusion in the prevention of early rebleeding following acute variceal hemorrhage in patients with cirrhosis. Variceal Bleeding Study Group. J Hepatol 1998;29:779–88.
33. Moitinho E, Planas R, Bañares R, et al. Multicenter randomized controlled trial comparing different schedules of somatostatin in the treatment of acute variceal bleeding. J Hepatol 2001;35:712–8.
34. Corley DA, Cello JP, Adkisson W, et al. Octreotide for acute esophageal variceal bleeding: a meta-analysis. Gastroenterology 2001;120:946–54.
35. Escorsell A, Bandi JC, Andreu V, et al. Desensitization to the effects of intravenous octreotide in cirrhotic patients with portal hypertension. Gastroenterology 2001;120:161–9.
36. Villanueva C, Colomo A, Aracil C, et al. Current endoscopic therapy for variceal bleeding. Best Pract Res Clin Gastroenterol 2008;22:261–78.
37. Park WG, Yeh RW, Triadafilopoulos G. Injection therapies for variceal bleeding disorders of the GI tract. Gastrointest Endosc 2008;67:313–23.
38. Baillie J, Yudelman P. Complications of endoscopic sclerotherapy of esophageal varices. Endoscopy 1992;24:284–91.
39. Lee JG, Lieberman DA. Complications related to endoscopic hemostasis techniques. Gastrointest Endosc Clin N Am 1996;6:305–21.
40. Rolando N, Gimson A, Philpott-Howard J, et al. Infectious sequelae after endoscopic sclerotherapy of oesophageal varices: role of antibiotic prophylaxis. J Hepatol 1993;18:290–4.
41. Selby WS, Norton ID, Pokorny CS, et al. Bacteremia and bacterascites after endoscopic sclerotherapy for bleeding esophageal varices and prevention by intravenous cefotaxime: a randomized trial. Gastrointest Endosc 1994;40:680–4.
42. Baron TH, Wong Kee Song LM. Endoscopic variceal band ligation. Am J Gastroenterol 2009;104:1083–5.
43. De Franchis R, Primignani M. Endoscopic treatments for portal hypertension. Semin Liver Dis 1999;19:439–55.
44. Stiegmann GV, Sun JH, Hammond WS. Results of experimental endoscopic esophageal varix ligation. Am Surg 1988;54:105–8.
45. Laine L, El-Newhi HM, Migikovsky B, et al. Endoscopic ligation compared with sclerotherapy for the treatment of bleeding esophageal varices. Ann Intern Med 1993;119:1–7.
46. Avgerinos A, Armonis A, Stefanidis G, et al. Sustained rise of portal pressure after sclerotherapy, but not band ligation, in acute variceal bleeding in cirrhosis. Hepatology 2004;39:1623–30.
47. Ramirez FC, Colon VJ, Landan D, et al. The effects of the number of rubber bands placed at each endoscopic session upon variceal outcomes: a prospective, randomized study. Am J Gastroenterol 2007;102:1372–6.
48. Shaheen NJ, Stuart E, Schmitz SM, et al. Pantoprazole reduces the size of postbanding ulcers after variceal band ligation: a randomized, controlled trial. Hepatology 2005;41:588–94.
49. Garcia-pagan JC, Bosch J. Endoscopic band ligation in the treatment of portal hypertension. Nat Clin Pract Gastroenterol Hepatol 2005;2:526–35.
50. D'Amico G, Pietrosi G, Tarantino I, et al. Emergency sclerotherapy versus vasoactive drugs for variceal bleeding in cirrhosis: a Cochrane meta-analysis. Gastroenterology 2003;124:1277–91.

51. Garcia-Tsao G, Sanyal AJ, Grace ND, et al. Prevention and management of gastroesophageal varices and variceal hemorrhage in cirrhosis. Hepatology 2007;46(3):922–38.
52. Villanueva C, Ortiz J, Sabat M, et al. Somatostatin alone or combined with emergency sclerotherapy in the treatment of acute esophageal variceal bleeding: a prospective randomized trial. Hepatology 1999;30(2):384–9.
53. Banares R, Albillos A, Rincon D, et al. Endoscopic treatment versus endoscopic plus pharmacologic treatment for acute variceal bleeding: a meta-analysis. Hepatology 2002;35:609–15.
54. Avgerinos A, Klonis C, Rekoumis G, et al. A prospective randomized trial comparing somatostatin, balloon tamponade and the combination of both methods in the management of acute variceal haemorrhage. J Hepatol 1991; 13:78–83.
55. Hubmann R, Bodlaj G, Czompo M, et al. The use of self-expanding metal stents to treat acute variceal bleeding. Endoscopy 2006;38:896–901.

Endoscopic Therapy for Gastric Varices

S.K. Sarin, MD, DM*, S.R. Mishra, MD, DM

KEYWORDS

- Gastric variceal bleeding • Cyanoacrylate
- Endoscopic therapy • Thrombin

Bleeding from gastric varices (GVs) is generally more severe than bleeding from esophageal varices (EVs),[1] but is thought to occur less frequently.[2–4] Although several recent developments in the agents and the techniques have improved the outcome of GV bleeds, no consensus has been reached on the optimum treatment. Because the blood flow in the GVs is relatively large and the bleeding is rapid and often profuse, endoscopic means of treating bleeding GVs are the treatments of choice. The choice of endoscopic therapy used often depends on local availability and expertise. In this article, the authors review the current endoscopic treatment modalities used in gastric variceal bleeding, and the primary and secondary prophylaxis of gastric variceal bleeding.

CLASSIFICATION OF GASTRIC VARICES

The endoscopic treatment modalities depend to a large extent on an accurate categorization of GVs The most widely used classification system is that proposed by the authors,[1] and this has been recommended for use by the Baveno consensus working group.[5] This classification categorizes GVs on the basis of their location in the stomach and their relationship with EVs (**Fig. 1**). Gastroesophageal varices (GOVs) are associated with varices along the lesser curve (type 1 [GOV1]), or along the fundus (type 2 [GOV2]); isolated gastric varices (IGVs) are present in isolation in the fundus (IGV1) or at ectopic sites in the stomach or the first part of the duodenum (IGV2). GOV1 are responsible for 70% of GVs, and can be managed as EVs. It is for the other types that the clinician is faced with several choices.

ENDOSCOPIC TREATMENT OF GASTRIC VARICES

Endoscopic treatment modalities available for gastric variceal bleed are:

1. Gastric variceal sclerotherapy (GVS)
2. Gastric variceal obturation (GVO) with glue

201, Academic Block, Department of Gastroenterology, G B Pant Hospital, University of Delhi, Institute of Liver and Biliary Sciences (ILBS), New Delhi, India
* Corresponding author.
E-mail address: shivsarin@gmail.com

Clin Liver Dis 14 (2010) 263–279
doi:10.1016/j.cld.2010.03.007
liver.theclinics.com

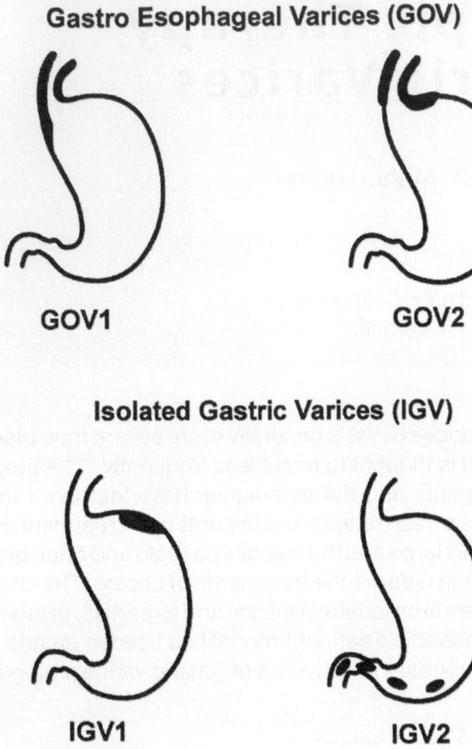

Fig. 1. Classification of GV.

3. Gastric variceal band ligation (GVL) with or without detachable snares
4. Thrombin injection (bovine or human)
5. Combined endoscopic therapy.

GASTRIC VARICEAL SCLEROTHERAPY

While endoscopic sclerotherapy has been effective in the treatment of EV bleeding and in eradication of EV,[2–4] it has been less successful in the management of GV, probably because of the high volume of blood flow through GV compared with EV, resulting in rapid flushing away of the sclerosant in the bloodstream. GVS typically requires larger volumes of sclerosant than for EV,[1,6] and fundal varices (GOV2 and IGV1) require significantly more sclerosant than GOV1.[7] This result may be associated with more side effects after GVS, such as fever, retrosternal and abdominal pain, and large ulcerations.[7] In acute GV bleeding, GVS has been reported to control bleeding in 60% to 100% of cases[3,7–9] (**Table 1**), but with unacceptably high rebleeding rates of up to 90%.[9,10] GVS appears to be least successful in controlling acute fundal variceal bleeding.[8,11] Differences observed between studies may reflect different injection techniques and different mixes of GV subtypes, but also inclusion of different patient populations; half of the patients in one study had noncirrhotic PHT,[12] whereas in the other studies more patients had cirrhosis. GVS achieved secondary prophylactic variceal eradication in 40% to 70% of all GV patients treated electively,[7,13] but the investigators found that this success was weighted heavily by high efficacy for GOV1 (95% eradication) and lower efficacy for GOV2 and IGV1. In that study, rebleeding after elective GVS was less than 20% for patients with GOV1 and GOV2 but it was high in

Table 1
Endoscopic sclerotherapy for gastric variceal bleeding

Authors	Agent	N	Success (%)	Rebleeding (%)	Complications
Trudeau and Prindiville, 1986[9]	STD	9	100	90	Ulcer 89%
Bretagne et al, 1986[10]	Polidocanol	10	60	63	–
Gimson et al, 1991[14]	EO/Glue	41	40	16	Ulcer 29% perforation
Oho et al, 1995[28]	EO (5%)	24	67	25	–
Chang et al, 1996[17]	STD (1.5%)	25	80	70	Ulcer 30%
Chang et al, 1996[83]	GW (50%)	26	92	30	Ulcer 30%
Sarin et al, 1997[12]	AA (95%)	18	67	34	Ulcer 100%
Ogawa et al, 1999[29]	EO (5%)	21	81	100	–
Sarin et al, 2002[13]	AA (95%)	8	62	25	–

Abbreviations: AA, absolute alcohol; EO, ethanol oleate; GW, glucose water; STD, sodium tetradecyl sulfate.

patients with IGV1 (53%).[7] Most bleeds were related to ulcers at the injection site, possibly related to the large amounts of sclerosant often needed in this situation. In an uncontrolled study of 41 patients, overall control of bleeding (44% vs 85%) and bleeding-related mortality (41% vs 8%) after sclerotherapy was worse for patients with bleeding fundal varices compared with GOV1.[14]

Following an index therapy for GV after a bleed, as part of an eradication program, repeat sclerotherapy is usually performed at 1- to 2-week intervals. Most of the studies (see **Table 1**) report high rebleeding rates of 50% to 90%.[4,6,7] Furthermore, in cirrhotic patients control of rebleeding episodes is significantly worse for GV than for EV.[9] Rebleeding appears to be worse for patients with bleeding fundal varices compared with GOV1 (77% vs 58%), probably reflecting the low rate of variceal eradication (24%).[14] These findings were reinforced by a large study of 71 patients (46% cirrhotic) in which patients with GOV2, and particularly IGV1, had lower rates of variceal obliteration (70% and 47%, respectively, vs 94% for GOV1) and a higher rate of rebleeding (19% and 53%, respectively, vs 6% for GOV1).[7]

The complication rates following sclerotherapy depend on local expertise and the frequency of follow-up, and vary between 19% and 82%.[13–16] Low-grade fever, retrosternal chest pain, temporary dysphagia, and asymptomatic pleural effusions occur commonly within the first 24 to 48 hours and usually do not require specific treatment.[15] Perforations and mediastinitis are complications that are more serious, and the latter results in mortality in excess of 50%. Mucosal ulcers are also commonly seen, and cause rebleeding.[13] Approximately 50% of rebleeding is caused by sclerotherapy-induced ulcers and is difficult to control, with a success rate between 9% and 44%.[9,17]

GVS is an effective and appropriate treatment for treatment of acute GOV1 hemorrhage and for attempting secondary prophylactic GOV1 obliteration. It is not appropriate for patients with fundal varices (GOV2 or IGV1) because of the low rate of primary hemostasis, the low success rate for secondary variceal eradication, and the high rate of rebleeding and complications.

GASTRIC VARICEAL OBTURATION

Obturation or obliteration is the term used for GVs treated by glue rather than eradication, as the varix itself can be visible even when it has been effectively treated. Tissue adhesive such as *N*-butyl-2-cyanoacrylate, which is a monomer that rapidly undergoes exothermic polymerization on contact with the hydroxyl ions present in water, has been used. The double bonds present in the monomer become single bonds, causing them to link together in enormous chains, changing the liquid to a hard brittle acrylic plastic.[18] Degradation occurs by hydrolysis, leading to the formation of smaller oligomers, and the production of formaldehyde, leading to possible histotoxicity.[19] Because of its rapid polymerization on contact with living tissues and its liquid consistency, cyanoacrylate has been used to eradicate and treat GVs. *N*-Butyl-2-cyanoacrylate is commonly used in Europe and Asia but is not available in the United States. However, a similar agent, 2-octyl cyanoacrylate, has been approved by the Food and Drug Administration in the United States for skin closure, and has also been used for the management of GVs.[20]

The technique for GVO has been standardized and should be carefully learnt. Eye protection is required during preparation and injection. A standard forward-viewing gastroscope is used, and its tip is coated with silicone or lipiodol to prevent sticking of the glue to the endoscope. The biopsy channel may be flushed with lubricant (such as silicone) to facilitate catheter insertion. A disposable steel-hubbed sclerotherapy injection needle, generally 21-gauge and at least 4 to 6 mm long, is selected. The catheter should be preloaded before insertion into the scope and should be primed with saline solution, followed by approximately 1 to 1.5 mL of undiluted cyanoacrylate (or a mixture of 1:1 cyanoacrylate and lipiodol)[21] to fill the dead space within the injection catheter. It is essential to know the volume of the dead space of the catheter used, which can be measured by prior injection of saline.

After puncturing the varix lumen with the needle, cyanoacrylate is injected in 1- to 1.5-mL aliquots by using normal saline or sterile water (about 0.8 to 1.0 mL, equal to the dead space) to flush the glue into the varix. As the needle is withdrawn from the varix, a steady stream of flush solution is aimed at the puncture site. The needle should be withdrawn immediately after the glue injection to prevent its impaction into the tissue adhesive. Once hemostasis is achieved, the endoscope is withdrawn with the needle withdrawn into the injector. The tip of the endoscope should be immediately cleaned after withdrawal from the patient, and silicone oil applied. Endoscopic suction should be avoided throughout the procedure. The obliteration of the varix is assessed by reinserting the endoscope and by blunt palpation with the injector or a catheter. Additional glue is injected until the varix is "hard" to palpation. On subsequent endoscopies, the patency of the varix is assessed by either blunt palpation or endoscopic ultrasound (EUS). Pulsed Doppler has also been used to assess patency by insertion of the probe through the biopsy channel of the scope.[22] This technique also offers the advantage of being able to locate the varix before treatment and facilitates quick assessment of the sclerosing effect, although the required probes are not yet widely available. Weeks to months after the injection, the mucosa overlying the glue cast sloughs off and the plug is extruded into the stomach. Most evidence for the use of cyanoacrylate in gastric variceal bleeding comes from series based in India, Japan, Europe, and the United States, which report good initial hemostasis rates of over 90% (**Table 2**).[21,23–27]

The efficacy of glue in comparison with sclerotherapy has been examined in 3 studies (**Table 3**). Oho and colleagues[28] performed a nonrandomized prospective study of 53 patients with acute gastric variceal bleeding. Glue achieved significantly better hemostasis (93% vs 67%). In a retrospective study, Ogawa and colleagues[29] found significantly better hemostasis with glue. Furthermore, in a randomized controlled trial by Sarin and colleagues,[13] there was a trend toward better hemostasis (89% vs 62%) with glue when compared with alcohol (n = 37).

Table 2
***N*-Butyl-2-cyanoacrylate for gastric varices**

Authors	Study Design	N	Follow-up (mo)	Hemostasis (%)	Rebleeding (%)	Mortality (%)
Seewald et al, 2008[38]	Retro	131	60	100	17	47
Belletrutti et al, 2008[45]	Retro	34	–	94	12	18
Fry et al, 2008[46]	Retro	33	9	88	15	18
Marques et al, 2008[47]	Pros	48	18	87	41	44
Cheng et al, 2007[48]	Retro	635	3–115	95	8	7
Mumtaz et al, 2007[49]	Retro	50	–	100	14	6
Joo et al, 2007[50]	Retro	85	24	98	29	31
Kim et al, 2006[51]	Pros	86	11	93	16	45
Noophun et al, 2005[53]	Retro	24	8.3	71	10	6
Mahadeva et al, 2003[40]	Retro	23	6	96	35	24
Greenwald et al, 2003[23]	Pilot	44	12	95	20	23
Sarin et al, 2002[13]	RCT	9	15.4	89	22	11
Dhiman et al, 2002[21]	Retro	18	31.6	100	10.3	NA
Akahoshi et al, 2002[54]	Retro	52	28.1	98.2	52	45
Lo et al, 2001[64]	RCT	31	14	87	31	9
Iwase et al, 2001[24]	Retro	37	31	100	16	43
Kind et al, 2000[25]	Retro	174	36	97	15.5	19.5
Huang et al, 2000[52]	Retro	90	13.2	100	23	39
Lee et al, 2000[42]	RCT	49	NA	95.7	44.7	NA
Ogawa et al, 1999[29]	Historical controls	17	60	100	7.6	82.5
Miyazaki et al, 1998[79]	Retro	6	51	83.3	NA	NA
D'Imperio et al, 1996[41]	Pros	22	NA	81	NA	3.7
Oho et al, 1995[28]	Pros	29	14	93	25	38
Ramond et al, 1986[26]	Retro	49	12	93	58	54

Abbreviations: NA, not available; Pros, prospective; RCT, randomized controlled trial; Retro, retrospective.

Several complications have been reported (mostly as case reports) in association with cyanoacrylate injection. These complications are mainly thrombotic in nature and include cerebral embolization and stroke, portal vein embolization, splenic infarction, coronary emboli, with a series demonstrating fatal and nonfatal pulmonary emboli in up to 5% of cases.[30–35] In addition, concerns of potential carcinogenesis have been raised in a study reporting the induction of sarcomas in the implantation site of rats injected with histoacryl.[36] Elective cyanoacrylate injection for nonbleeding GVs is not associated with significant bacteremia or infection, and prophylactic antibiotics may not be needed in this patient group. By contrast, prophylactic antibiotics are

Table 3
Gastric variceal sclerotherapy versus glue injection for gastric variceal bleeding

Authors	Agent	N	Hemostasis (%)	Rebleeding (%)	Ulcer (%)	Mortality (%)
Oho et al, 1995[28]	EO	24	67	12.5	25	67
	HC	29	93	10	30	38
Ogawa et al, 1999[29]	EO	21	81	35	–	23.8
	HC	17	100	0		0
Sarin et al, 2002[13]	AA	8	62	25	82	25
	HC	9	89	22	65	11

Abbreviation: HC, histoacryl.

strongly recommended for patients with bleeding GVs undergoing cyanoacrylate injection.[37] GVO requires some skill and care to prevent damage to equipment, and caution is required in view of the reported embolic phenomena.[38]

Even in young infants, the use of cyanoacrylate glue is safe and effective for the treatment of gastric variceal bleed.[39] In a retrospective analysis, Mahadeva and colleagues[40] retrospectively analyzed that cyanoacrylate glue injection was more cost effective than transjugular intrahepatic portosystemic shunt (TIPSS) in the management of acute gastric variceal bleeding. A prospective, randomized trial would be required to confirm this observation. Use of undiluted cyanoacrylate was shown to be safe and effective and also to be associated with fewer complications, in contrast to the diluted form.[21,41] The authors prefer the undiluted form of cyanoacrylate, which is efficacious and safe for controlling acute GV bleeding and for preventing GV rebleeding.

To prevent rebleeding, twice-weekly EUS-guided obliteration was compared with "on demand" treatment (given in response to rebleeding) in an uncontrolled study of 101 cirrhotic patients. Late rebleeding (>48 hours) was significantly less in the EUS group (19% vs 45%), even though the incidence of postinjection ulcers was significantly higher in the EUS group.[42] The overall rate of variceal eradication was 80% for GOV1, GOV2, and IGV1. In a small case series, EUS-guided injection of cyanoacrylate at the level of the perforating veins in the treatment of GVs was found to be safe, efficient, and perhaps an accurate approach.[43] Linhares and colleagues[44] use fluoroscopic guidance for injection of cyanoacrylate, which seems to be safe and effective for assessing proper obturation of gastric varices.

Several recent long-term studies also reported hemostasis rates of 90% and low rebleeding rates of 15% to 30% with cyanoacrylate injection, with 1 to 3 injections needed to achieve obliteration, with higher eradication rates for GOV1 and GOV2 than IGV1.[45–54]

At present it is clear that GVO using tissue adhesives has high efficacy and safety for the control of acute GV bleed and for the prevention of GV rebleeding, and is the treatment of choice.[5,55] However, to prevent rebleeding other methods and devices are being evaluated. In 2 recent prospective randomized trials, cyanoacrylate injection was compared with TIPSS[56] and balloon-occluded retrograde transvenous obliteration (BRTO)[57] in gastric variceal bleeding. Lo and colleagues[56] showed that TIPS is more effective than glue injection in preventing rebleeding from GVs, with a similar survival and frequency of complications. Hong and colleagues[57] showed that the therapeutic efficacy of cyanoacrylate and BRTO for the treatment of active GV bleed and/or high-risk GV appeared to be similar; however, cyanoacrylate might be associated with a higher rebleeding rate than BRTO, and the investigators suggested BRTO could be an effective rescue treatment for patients with GV bleed after initial treatment with cyanoacrylate.

In a recently completed randomized controlled trial (S.K. Sarin and S.R. Mishra, unpublished data, 2006–2009), the authors evaluated the role of endoscopic cyanoacrylate injection (n = 32) in patients with fundal varices (GOV2 with eradicated esophageal varix and IGV1) who had bled before, comparing it with β-blocker therapy (n = 32). The actuarial probability of GV bleeding-free rate in the cyanoacrylate group was significantly higher than that of the β-blocker group (85% vs 45%, $P = .004$), and the mortality rate was lower (3% vs 25%, $P = .026$) during a median follow-up of 24 months. There were no serious adverse events observed with endoscopic cyanoacrylate injection during the study period. The authors conclude that cyanoacrylate injection is more effective than β-blocker therapy for the prevention of GV rebleeding and improving survival.

GASTRIC VARICEAL BAND LIGATION

Variceal band ligation is an established treatment for the prevention of esophageal variceal bleeding and rebleeding. Early attempts at ligating GVs using detachable snares and "O" rings were promising, although there is a lack of controlled clinical trials. Current methods involve the use of a multiband device such as the 6-Shooter Multi-Band Ligator.[58] This instrument can be used in actively bleeding varices after initial identification of the bleeding varix. Banding in both retroflexed and nonretroflexed positions may be performed. It is not usually necessary to apply more than 4 bands in one session.[58] EVs, if present, should also be banded in the same session, starting at the gastroesophageal junction. A further development was the use of the detachable snare for GVs larger than 2 cm and elastic bands for smaller varices.[59] In this study of 41 cirrhotic patients with predominantly cardiac varices and recent hemorrhage (12 actively bleeding), there was an 83% rate of initial hemostasis. Others have reported 100% hemostasis with the use of a detachable snare, although only 8 patients with active bleeding were included in this study.[60]

In 5 uncontrolled studies[58,60–63] (**Table 4**), active GV bleed was controlled with 100% success with a very low rebleeding rate of 10%–20%, and also the GV was obliterated in all cases. In the recently published study by Lee and Shih,[63] the early rebleeding was still a problem and was more often encountered with larger GVs.

GVL has been compared with tissue adhesives in 2 randomized controlled studies (**Table 5**).[64,65] In the first study, cirrhotics were randomized to either butyl cyanoacrylate injection (n = 31, mean follow-up 14 months) or GVL (n = 29, mean follow-up 9 months).[64] Most patients had GOV1 (69%) followed by GOV2 (24%) and IGV1 (7%). There were 26 patients with active bleeding, and 34 with stigmata of recent hemorrhage. Initial hemostasis was significantly better in the cyanoacrylate group (87% vs

Table 4
Gastric variceal ligation in the management of gastric variceal bleeding

Author	Therapy	N	Active Bleed (%)	Success (%)	Rebleeding (%)	Obliteration (%)
Yoshida et al, 1994[84]	GVL-S	10	10	100	10	100
Harada et al, 1997[61]	GVL-S	5	100	100	20	–
Cipolletta et al, 1998[62]	GVL-S	7	100	100	0	–
Shiha and El Sayed, 1999[58]	GVL	27	67	89	18	100
Lee and Shih, 2008[63]	GVL	22	100	100	18	–

Abbreviation: GVL-S, gastric variceal ligation – sclerotherapy.

Table 5
Variceal band ligation versus tissue adhesives

Authors	Treatment	Study Type	N (Follow-up)	Active bleeding (%)	Hemostasis (%)	Rebleeding (%)	Mortality (%)
Lo et al, 2001[64]	HO/VBL	RCT	29/31 (12 mo)	43	87/45	31/54	48/29 ($P = .05$)
Tan et al, 2006[65]	HO/VBL	RCT	49/48 (23/20 mo)	31	93/93	22/44	55/69

Abbreviation: HO, histoacryl.

45%), with one patient being rescued by glue injection after failure of banding. There were no significant differences in bleeding-related deaths. The second large study comprised 97 patients with cirrhosis.[65] The differences in this study are a longer follow-up of almost 2 years and a greater proportion of patients with IGV1. A total of 31 patients presented with acute bleeding, and hemostasis was achieved in more than 90% with both modalities. The investigators attributed the better efficacy of GVL than the previous study[64] to a greater number of bands used (4.5 vs 1–2 bands), although there was no difference in bleed-related mortality. The trial is noteworthy for being the largest controlled study in patients with GV bleed,[65] and illustrates that good technique of GVL can significantly influence outcome.

The evidence for the use of GVL for acute gastric variceal bleeding is mixed, and at best GVL is a second alternative therapy to tissue adhesives. Although initial hemostasis may be achieved with GVL, the main disadvantage has been high rate of rebleeding, probably from feeding vessels. Repeat endoscopy and variceal band ligation (VBL) is thus necessary at 1- to 2-weekly intervals until eradication of varices or until only small residual varices remain. Some investigators have used mucosal protectors such as sucralfate to aid healing of banding-induced ulcers.[64] Others have used detachable snares to eradicate large GVs in cirrhotic patients, with good results, although the follow-up period was very short (3.8 months).[62] Use of a detachable snare for GVs larger than 2 cm and elastic bands for smaller varices followed by propranolol after eradication led to a low rebleeding rate of 11%.[59] However, the cumulative variceal recurrence rate was 100% at 2 years.

The randomized trials by Lo and colleagues[64] and Tan and colleagues[65] mentioned earlier, comparing histoacryl injection and VBL, reported worse outcome for secondary prevention in the VBL arm, with almost twice the rebleeding rate.[64,65] The therapies were performed at 3- to 4-weekly intervals, with 2 to 3 sessions required in each treatment arm to eradicate varices. The rates of eradication of varices and overall mortality were similar. Outcomes were similar for all types of GVs in the former study, although Tan and colleagues showed that the benefit of tissue adhesives was particularly evident with IGV1. For secondary prophylaxis of GV bleed, injection of tissue adhesives is preferred over GVL. The use of detachable snares or combination therapy with sclerotherapy may give better results, but controlled trials are lacking and therefore, these newer techniques cannot be recommended for routine clinical practice.

THROMBIN

Thrombin is a hemostatic agent that was first used for the management of GVs in 1947.[66] There have been subsequent uncontrolled studies using thrombin for both esophageal and GV bleeding (**Table 6**).[67–75] Some studies have also investigated the use of thrombin in combination with sclerosing agents.[67] Thrombin is commercially available as a sterile, lypophilized powder. Thrombin principally affects hemostasis by converting fibrinogen to a fibrin clot. Initially, thrombin catalyzes the conversion of fibrinogen to fibrinogen monomers. These monomers spontaneously aggregate, forming a weak fibrin clot. Thrombin also converts factors XIII to XIIIa, which converts these monomers to a cross-linked fibrin polymer. Thrombin has other effects on hemostasis such as platelet aggregation. In rare cases where there is a primary clotting disorder resulting in the absence of fibrinogen, thrombin will fail to clot blood. A 5-mL solution of thrombin containing 1000 units/mL of thrombin will clot a liter of blood in less than 60 seconds. In a patient with bleeding GV, thrombin is reconstituted and 1 mL aliquot is injected into the bleeding varix. The needle should only be exposed when the outer sheath is next to the varix, to minimize the risk of inadvertent injection of thrombin in the surrounding mucosa.

Bovine Thrombin

Only small series of patients have reported the use of thrombin injection. Initial studies by Williams and colleagues[68] in an uncontrolled series of 11 consecutive patients using bovine thrombin resulted in 100% success of initial control of gastric variceal bleeding. The patients had predominantly viral hepatitis, and bleeding fundal varices. The average dose of thrombin required for each patient was 5.5 mL (5500 U/mL) per session. There were no complications related to the procedure or thromboembolic events. In another study published in abstract form, bovine thrombin injections achieved hemostasis in 96% of patients who had gastric and esophageal variceal bleeding refractory to injection sclerotherapy.[69] Przemioslo and colleagues[70] studied bovine thrombin in 52 patients who presented with bleeding GVs (63%), or bleeding from both GVs and EVs (37%). The average dose of thrombin used was 10.7 mL (100 IU/mL) for the first session. Bleeding EVs were treated with thrombin sclerotherapy and VBL. Initial hemostasis was achieved in 94% of patients. There were no complications reported. Recently, Ramesh and colleagues[71] showed that endoscopic treatment of bovine thrombin is effective in 92% of patients with bleeding GVs, without any rebleeding in a follow-up period of almost 2 years. The small number of cases, retrospective nature, and uncontrolled study are the limitations.

Human Thrombin

Yang and colleagues[72] retrospectively evaluated the use of human thrombin in 12 patients with GV bleeding. Immediate hemostasis was achieved in all patients in whom there was active bleeding from GVs at the time of endoscopy (n = 6). There were no immediate allergic reactions, thromboembolic complications, or rebleeding. There have been 2 uncontrolled series that evaluated the role of Beriplast-P (human thrombin) in patients with bleeding GV. This preparation differs from that used by Yang and colleagues in that it is composed of 2 separate constituents, the first containing fibrinogen and factor XIII and the second containing human thrombin. The constituents are injected into the bleeding varix through a double-lumen syringe, immediately forming a fibrin clot. Heneghan and colleagues[73] studied 10 patients presenting with acute GV bleeding. A median dose of 6 mL was used. The results appeared promising, with immediate hemostasis achieved in 70% patients and with no patient having rebled from GVs over a follow-up period of 8 months. However, 5 patients (50%) rebled from EVs, and the overall mortality rate was alarmingly high at 50%, principally from variceal bleeding and multiorgan failure. Therefore, the overall outcome is unfavorable despite the efficacy in treating GV bleeding. The second study

Table 6
Thrombin in bleeding GVs

Authors	Treatment	N	Follow-up (mo)	Hemostasis (%)	Variceal Recurrence (%)	Rebleeding (%)	Mortality (%)
Kitano et al, 1989[67]	ES/TM + ES	25/25	–	–	–	54/6	4/4
Williams et al, 1994[68]	TM	11	9	100	0	27	0
Przemioslo et al, 1999[70]	TM	52	1.5	94	16	18	8
Snobl et al, 1992[69]	TM	72	–	96	–	–	–
Yang et al, 2002[72]	TM	12	17	100	–	25	17
Heneghan et al, 2002[73]	TM	10	8	70	–	50	50
Datta et al, 2003[74]	TM	15	1	93	–	28	7
Ramesh et al, 2008[71]	TM	13	25	92	–	7	38

Abbreviations: ES, endoscopic sclerotherapy; TM, thrombin.

involved 15 patients, with a very short follow-up of 30 days.[74] The volume of Beriplast used was 4.5 to 6 mL, with the higher volume used for fundal varices. Initial hemostasis was achieved in 14 patients, and the 30-day mortality was 7%, as there were fewer patients with advanced liver disease than in the former study.[73] There were no complications related to the procedure or systemic activation of the clotting system, such as distant embolization. Thrombin was used successfully in 4 patients in whom attempts at TIPSS insertion were unsuccessful, suggesting a role for thrombin in patients for whom conventional treatments had failed. These findings have been supported by a retrospective series involving 33 patients, where 100% hemostasis was achieved.[75]

Thrombin has not been subjected to controlled studies, and is not universally accepted for secondary prophylaxis. Human thrombin in combination with 5% ethanolamine was used by Kitano and colleagues[67] in a prospective randomized trial for bleeding varices. Results were encouraging, with lower rebleeding rates achieved in the thrombin plus sclerosant arm compared with sclerosant alone (6% vs 54%). There were higher levels of fibrin degradation products in the thrombin arm, but no clinical complications were noted. The study was limited by a short follow-up time and the absence of a thrombin monotherapy arm. The study by Yang and colleagues[72] reported a rebleeding rate of 25% over an average of 17.8 months. In the larger series reported in an abstract form, the rebleeding rate was only 11%, even though eradication was achieved in only 6%.[75] These results highlight the potential for thrombin to be used "on demand" as opposed to elective variceal eradication; further studies comparing the 2 approaches would be invaluable. Of the 2 studies using Berilplast-P,[73,74] only one offered repeat injections electively or at the time of rebleeding.[74] This study reported a rebleeding rate of 29%. The limited evidence for bovine thrombin showed rebleeding rates of 27%[68] and 18%,[70] with 1 to 3 sessions required for variceal eradication.

Thrombin seems to be a promising therapy, and has the benefits of achieving excellent initial hemostasis and being easy to use with a good safety profile. Thrombin appears to be successful even in patients with GOV2, and may have a role in this difficult group. Further controlled studies comparing it with other treatment modalities are required before it can be universally recommended.[76]

COMBINED ENDOSCOPIC THERAPY

Combined endoscopic methods in the setting of acute GV bleed have been studied for the control of bleeding and to prevent rebleeding (**Table 7**). Chun and Hyun[77] showed that endoscopic variceal ligation-injection sclerotherapy (EVLIS) is safe and effective in achieving hemostasis and obliteration in all patients. Takeuchi and colleagues[78] and Lee and colleagues[42] performed GVL with snare, where the success rate in controlling acute GV bleed was 83% to 93%, with a lower rebleeding rate (2%–10%). In 16 patients with GV, Miyazaki and colleagues[79] showed that combined injection sclerotherapy using *N*-butyl-2-cyanoacrylate and ethanolamine oleate was a safe and useful treatment, but 57% of patients had a rebleed. A larger uncontrolled study in 56 cirrhotic patients with GOV1 (67%) and IGV1 (33%) type varices used a combination of GVL with "O" rings and sclerotherapy.[80] Using this technique, GVs were banded with "O" rings (mean of 1–9 bands, more for large varices in cardia and fundus). Then 1% polidocanol was injected in the surrounding submucosa (mean volume 55 mL). There was 100% hemostasis in the 18 patients with active bleeding. This laborious therapy resulted in a low rate of variceal bleeding of 8% at 2 years, without serious complications, and excellent rates of variceal eradication with a 2-year recurrence rate of 15%.[80] Combination of variceal ligation and cyanoacrylate injection in GV effectively controlled acute bleed in 89% of patients; however 33% rebled on follow-up.[81] After

Table 7
Combined endoscopic modalities

References	Therapy	N	Acute Bleeding (%)	Success (%)	Rebleeding (%)	Obliteration (%)
Chun and Hyun, 1995[77]	GVL EIS	32	33	100	0	100
Takeuchi et al, 1996[78]	GVL GVL-S	45	13	83	2	94
Miyazaki, 1998[79]	EIS EST-NBC	16	37	83	57	43
Yoshida et al, 1999[60]	GVL-S EISL	35	23	100	8	97
Lee et al, 2002[42]	GVL-S GVL-B	41	30	92.7	10.5	91.7
Arakaki et al, 2003[80]	GVL-B EST	56	32	100	3.6	100
Sugimoto et al, 2007[81]	GVL-B EST-NBC	27	–	88.9	33	–

Abbreviations: EIS, endoscopic injection sclerotherapy; EISL, endoscopic injection sclerotherapy and ligation; EST, endoscopic sclerotherapy; GVL-B, gastric variceal ligation – banding; NBC, N butyl-2-cyanoacrylate.

successful obliteration of bleeding GVs with Histoacryl (n = 67), Kuo and colleagues[82] divided them into 2 groups: a combined group of patients who had adjuvant injection of hypertonic glucose solutions in cases of residual gastric varices (F1 or less) and a control group of patients who did not receive such therapy. Adjuvant treatment with hypertonic glucose solution for residual small GVs was found to be safe and to reduce the recurrence or progression of gastric varices (7% vs 29%, $P = .029$) after tissue adhesive injections. These studies on combined endoscopic therapy need further validation.

Combination with sclerotherapy is unlikely to be accepted for the management of acute bleeding in view of the increased risk of iatrogenic complications, and the need for greater technical skill and procedure time. For secondary prophylaxis, combined therapy should be compared with standard established treatments.

PRIMARY PROPHYLAXIS FOR GASTRIC VARICEAL BLEEDING

There are limited data on the use of therapies for primary prophylaxis, but treatments may have the greatest role for large IGV1 and GOV2 where there is a high risk of bleeding. There are not enough data to recommend any particular endoscopic therapy. It is important to consider iatrogenic complications, such as ulcers and embolization, with tissue adhesives. In a recently completed randomized controlled trial (S.K. Sarin and S.R. Mishra, unpublished data, 2006–2009), the authors evaluated the role of endoscopic cyanoacrylate injection (n = 25) in patients with GV (GOV2 with eradicated esophageal varix and IGV1) who had never bled before, comparing it with β-blocker therapy (n = 24) and a third arm that did not receive treatment for GVs (n = 25). In the cyanoacrylate group, 8% of patients bled and in the β-blocker group 33% of patients bled, in contrast to 48% of patients in the no-treatment group (cyanoacrylate group vs no treatment group [$P = .022$], cyanoacrylate group vs β-blocker group [$P = .042$])

over a median follow-up of 24 months. One (4%) patient in the cyanoacrylate group and 8 (25%) patients in the no treatment group died ($P = .046$). There were no serious adverse events observed with endoscopic cyanoacrylate injection during the study period. The authors concluded that endoscopic cyanoacrylate injection is safe, prevented gastric variceal bleeding, and improved the survival in patients who had never previously bled from GV (GOV2 and IGV1).

SUMMARY

GOV1 should be treated just like EVs. For fundal varices, various endoscopic methods of treatment are available. Tissue adhesives are the first line of therapy for the control of acute GV bleeding and prevention of GV rebleeding. Endoscopic sclerotherapy is less efficacious in achieving hemostasis, with high rebleeding rate and high incidence of local complications. VBL is an alternative method to tissue adhesives. Thrombin is effective and very safe for the control of GV bleeding and is easy to use; however, controlled trials are required to establish its role.

REFERENCES

1. Sarin SK, Lahoti D, Saxena SP, et al. Prevalence, classification and natural history of gastric varices: a long-term follow-up study in 568 portal hypertension patients. Hepatology 1992;16:1343–9.
2. Paquet KJ, Feusener H. Endoscopic sclerosis and esophageal balloon tamponade in acute hemorrhage from esophagogastric varices. Hepatology 1985;5: 580–3.
3. Stray N, Jacobsen CD, Rosseland A. Injection sclerotherapy of bleeding oesophageal and gastric varices using a flexible endoscope. Acta Med Scand 1982;211:125–9.
4. Jalan R, Hayes PC. UK guidelines on the management of variceal haemorrhage in cirrhotic patients. British Society of Gastroenterology. Gut 2000;46(Suppl 3–4): III1–III15.
5. de Franchis R. Evolving consensus in Portal Hypertension Report of the Baveno IV Consensus Workshop on methodology of diagnosis and therapy in portal hypertension. J Hepatol 2005;43:167–76.
6. Sarin SK, Lahoti D. Management of gastric varices. Baillieres Clin Gastroenterol 1992;6:527–48.
7. Sarin SK. Long-term follow-up of gastric variceal sclerotherapy: an eleven-year experience. Gastrointest Endosc 1997;46:8–14.
8. Korula J, Chin K, Ko Y, et al. Demonstration of two distinct subsets of gastric varices. Observations during a seven-year study of endoscopic sclerotherapy. Dig Dis Sci 1991;36:303–9.
9. Trudeau W, Prindiville T. Endoscopic injection sclerosis in bleeding gastric varices. Gastrointest Endosc 1986;32:264–8.
10. Bretagne JF, Dudicourt JC, Morisot D, et al. Is endoscopic variceal sclerotherapy effective for the treatment of gastric varices [abstract]. Dig Dis Sci 1986; 31:505S.
11. Millar AJ, Brown RA, Hill ID, et al. The fundal pile: bleeding gastric varices. J Pediatr Surg 1991;26:707–9.
12. Sarin SK, Govil A, Jain AK, et al. Prospective randomized trial of endoscopic sclerotherapy versus variceal band ligation for esophageal varices: influence on gastropathy, gastric varices and variceal recurrence. J Hepatol 1997;26:826–32.

13. Sarin SK, Jain AK, Jain M, et al. A randomized controlled trial of cyanoacrylate versus alcohol injection in patients with isolated fundic varices. Am J Gastroenterol 2002;97:1010–5.
14. Gimson AE, Westaby D, Williams R. Endoscopic sclerotherapy in the management of gastric variceal haemorrhage. J Hepatol 1991;13:274–8.
15. Schuman BM, Beckman JW, Tedesco FJ, et al. Complications of endoscopic injection sclerotherapy: a review. Am J Gastroenterol 1987;82:823–30.
16. Sarin SK, Lamba GS, Kumar M, et al. Comparison of endoscopic ligation and propranolol for the primary prevention of variceal bleeding. N Engl J Med 1999;340:988–93.
17. Chang KY, Wu CS, Chen PC. Prospective randomized trial of hypertonic glucose water and sodium tetradecyl sulfate for gastric variceal bleeding in patients with advanced liver cirrhosis. Endoscopy 1996;28:481–6.
18. Bloomfield L. Working knowledge: instant glue. Sci Am 1999;280:104.
19. Vinters HV, Galil KA, Lundie MJ, et al. The histotoxicity of cyanoacrylates. A selective review. Neuroradiology 1985;27:279–91.
20. Rengstorff DS, Binmoeller KF. A pilot study of 2-octyl cyanoacrylate injection for treatment of gastric fundal varices in humans. Gastrointest Endosc 2004;59: 553–8.
21. Dhiman RK, Chawla Y, Taneja S, et al. Endoscopic sclerotherapy of gastric variceal bleeding with N-butyl-2-cyanoacrylate. J Clin Gastroenterol 2002;35: 222–7.
22. Battaglia G, Bocus P, Morbin T, et al. Endoscopic Doppler US-guided injection therapy for gastric varices: case report. Gastrointest Endosc 2003;57:608–11.
23. Greenwald BD, Caldwell SH, Hespenheide EE, et al. N-2-butyl-cyanoacrylate for bleeding gastric varices: a United States pilot study and cost analysis. Am J Gastroenterol 2003;98:1982–8.
24. Iwase H, Maeda O, Shimada M, et al. Endoscopic ablation with cyanoacrylate glue for isolated gastric variceal bleeding. Gastrointest Endosc 2001;53:585–92.
25. Kind R, Guglielmi A, Rodella L, et al. Bucrylate treatment of bleeding gastric varices: 12 years' experience. Endoscopy 2000;32:512–9.
26. Ramond MJ, Valla D, Mosnier JF, et al. Successful endoscopic obturation of gastric varices with butyl cyanoacrylate. Hepatology 1989;10:488–93.
27. Sheikh RA, Trudeau WL. Clinical evaluation of endoscopic injection sclerotherapy using N-butyl-2-cyanoacrylate for gastric variceal bleeding. Gastrointest Endosc 2000;52:142–4.
28. Oho K, Iwao T, Sumino M, et al. Ethanolamine oleate vs. butyl cyanoacrylate for bleeding gastric varices: a nonrandomized study. Endoscopy 1995;27:349–54.
29. Ogawa K, Ishikawa S, Naritaka Y, et al. Clinical evaluation of endoscopic injection sclerotherapy using N-butyl-2-cyanoacrylate for gastric variceal bleeding. J Gastroenterol Hepatol 1999;14:245–50.
30. Roesch W, Rexroth G. Pulmonary, cerebral and coronary emboli during bucrylate injection of bleeding fundic varices. Endoscopy 1998;30:S89–90.
31. Huang SS, Kim HH, Park SH, et al. N-butyl-2-cyanoacrylate pulmonary embolism after endoscopic injection sclerotherapy for gastric variceal bleeding. J Comput Assist Tomogr 2001;25:16–22.
32. Palejwala AA, Smart HL, Hughes M. Multiple pulmonary glue emboli following gastric variceal obliteration. Endoscopy 2000;32:S1–2.
33. Yu LK, Hsu CW, Tseng JH, et al. Splenic infarction complicated by splenic artery occlusion after N-butyl-2-cyanoacrylate injection for gastric varices: case report. Gastrointest Endosc 2005;61:343–5.

34. Hamad N, Stephens J, Maskell GF, et al. Case report: thromboembolic and septic complications of migrated cyanoacrylate injection for bleeding gastric varices. Br J Radiol 2008;81:e263–5.
35. Marion-Audibert AM, Schoeffler M, Wallet F, et al. Acute pulmonary embolism during cyanoacrylate injection in gastric varices. Gastroenterol Clin Biol 2008; 32(11):926–30.
36. Reiter A. [Induction of sarcomas by the tissue-binding substance histoacryl-blau in the rat]. Z Exp Chir Transplant Kunstliche Organe 1987;20:55–60 [in German].
37. Rerknimitr R, Chanyaswad J, Kongkam P, et al. Risk of bacteremia in bleeding and nonbleeding gastric varices after endoscopic injection of cyanoacrylate. Endoscopy 2008;40:644–9.
38. Seewald S, Ang TL, Imazu H, et al. A standardized injection technique and regimen ensures success and safety of N-butyl-2-cyanoacrylate for the treatment of gastric fundal varices (with videos). Gastrointest Endosc 2008;68:447–54.
39. Rivet C, Robles-Medranda C, Dumortier J, et al. Endoscopic treatment of gastro-esophageal varices in young infants with cyanoacrylate glue: a pilot study. Gastrointest Endosc 2009;69(6):1034–8.
40. Mahadeva S, Bellamy MC, Kessel D, et al. Cost-effectiveness of N-butyl-2-cyano-acrylate (histoacryl) glue injections versus transjugular intrahepatic portosystemic shunt in the management of acute gastric variceal bleeding. Am J Gastroenterol 2003;98:2688–93.
41. D'Imperio N, Piemontese A, Baroncini D, et al. Evaluation of undiluted N-butyl-2-cyanoacrylate in the endoscopic treatment of upper gastrointestinal tract varices. Endoscopy 1996;28(2):239–43.
42. Lee YT, Chan FK, Ng EK, et al. EUS guided injection of cyanoacrylate for bleeding gastric varices. Gastrointest Endosc 2000;52:168–74.
43. Romero-Castro R, Pellicer-Bautista FJ, Jimenez-Saenz M, et al. EUS-guided injection of cyanoacrylate perforating feeding veins in gastric varices: results in 5 cases. Gastrointest Endosc 2007;66:402–7.
44. Linhares MM, Matone J, Matos D, et al. Endoscopic treatment of bleeding gastric varices using large amount of N-butyl-2-cyanoacrylate under fluoroscopic guidance. Surg Laparosc Endosc Percutan Tech 2008;18:441–4.
45. Belletrutti PJ, Romagnuolo J, Hilsden RJ, et al. Endoscopic management of gastric varices: efficacy and outcomes of gluing with N-butyl-2-cyanoacrylate in a North American patient population. Can J Gastroenterol 2008;22:931–6.
46. Fry LC, Neumann H, Olano C, et al. Efficacy, complications and clinical outcomes of endoscopic sclerotherapy with N-butyl-2-cyanoacrylate for bleeding gastric varices. Dig Dis 2008;26:300–3.
47. Marques P, Maluf-Filho F, Kumar A, et al. Long-term outcomes of acute gastric variceal bleeding in 48 patients following treatment with cyanoacrylate. Dig Dis Sci 2008;53:544–50.
48. Cheng LF, Wang ZQ, Li CZ, et al. Treatment of gastric varices by endoscopic sclerotherapy using butyl cyanoacrylate: 10 years experience of 635 cases. Chin Med J (Engl) 2007;120:2081–5.
49. Mumtaz K, Majid S, Shah H, et al. Prevalence of gastric varices and results of sclerotherapy with N-butyl 2 cyanoacrylate for controlling acute gastric variceal bleeding. World J Gastroenterol 2007;13:1247–51.
50. Joo HS, Jang JY, Eun SH, et al. Long-term results of endoscopic (N-butyl 2 cyanoacrylate) injection for treatment of gastric varices—a 10 years experience. Korean J Gastroenterol 2007;49:320–6.

51. Kim JW, Baik SK, Kim KH, et al. Effect of endoscopic sclerotherapy using N-butyl-2-cyanoacrylate in patients with gastric variceal bleeding. Korean J Hepatol 2006;12(3):394–403.
52. Huang YH, Yeh HZ, Chen GH, et al. Endoscopic treatment of bleeding gastric varices by N-butyl-2-cyanoacrylate (Histoacryl) injection: long-term efficacy and safety. Gastrointest Endosc 2000;52:160–7.
53. Noophun P, Kongkam P, Gonlachanvit S, et al. Bleeding gastric varices: results of endoscopic injection with cyanoacrylate at King Chulalongkorn Memorial Hospital. World J Gastroenterol 2005;11:7531–5.
54. Akahoshi T, Hashizume M, Shimabukuro R, et al. Long-term results of endoscopic histoacryl injection sclerotherapy for gastric variceal bleeding: a 10-year experience. Surgery 2002;131:S176–81.
55. Consolo P, Luigiano C, Giacobbe G, et al. Cyanoacrylate glue in the management of gastric varices. Minerva Med 2009;100(1):115–21.
56. Lo GH, Liang HL, Chen WC, et al. A prospective, randomized controlled trial of transjugular intrahepatic portosystemic shunt versus cyanoacrylate injection in the prevention of gastric variceal rebleeding. Endoscopy 2007;39(8):679–85.
57. Hong CH, Kim HJ, Park JH, et al. Treatment of patients with gastric variceal hemorrhage: endoscopic N-butyl-2-cyanoacrylate injection versus balloon-occluded retrograde transvenous obliteration. J Gastroenterol Hepatol 2009;24(3):372–8.
58. Shiha G, El Sayed SS. Gastric variceal ligation: a new technique. Gastrointest Endosc 1999;49:437–41.
59. Lee MS, Cho JY, Cheon YK, et al. Use of detachable snares and elastic bands for endoscopic control of bleeding from large gastric varices. Gastrointest Endosc 2002;56:83–8.
60. Yoshida T, Harada T, Shigemitsu T, et al. Endoscopic management of gastric varices using a detachable snare and simultaneous endoscopic sclerotherapy and O-ring ligation. J Gastroenterol Hepatol 1999;14:730–5.
61. Harada T, Yoshida T, Shigemitsu T, et al. Therapeutic results of endoscopic variceal ligation for acute bleeding of oesophageal and gastric varices. J Gastroenterol Hepatol 1997;12(4):331–5.
62. Cipolletta L, Bianco MA, Rotondano G, et al. Emergency endoscopic ligation of actively bleeding gastric varices with a detachable snare. Gastrointest Endosc 1998;47:400–3.
63. Lee TH, Shih LN. Clinical experience of endoscopic banding ligation for bleeding gastric varices. Hepatogastroenterology 2008;55:766–9.
64. Lo GH, Lai KH, Cheng JS, et al. A prospective, randomized trial of butyl cyanoacrylate injection vs. band ligation in the management of bleeding gastric varices. Hepatology 2001;33:1060–4.
65. Tan PC, Hou MC, Lin HC, et al. A randomized trial of endoscopic treatment of acute gastric variceal hemorrhage: N-butyl-2-cyanoacrylate injection vs. band ligation. Hepatology 2006;43:690–7.
66. Daly PM. Use of buffer thrombin in treatment of gastric varices: a preliminary report. Arch Surg 1947;55:208–12.
67. Kitano S, Hashizume M, Yamaga H, et al. Human thrombin plus 5 per cent ethanolamine oleate injected to sclerose oesophageal varices: a prospective randomized trial. Br J Surg 1989;76:715–8.
68. Williams SG, Peters RA, Westaby D. Thrombin—an effective treatment for gastric variceal haemorrhage. Gut 1994;35:1287–9.

69. Snobl J, Van Buuren HR, Van Blankenstein M. Endoscopic injection using thrombin: an effective and safe method for controlling oesophagogastric variceal bleeding [abstract]. Gastroenterology 1992;102:A891.
70. Przemioslo RT, McNair A, Williams R. Thrombin is effective in arresting bleeding from gastric variceal hemorrhage. Dig Dis Sci 1999;44:778–81.
71. Ramesh J, Limdi JK, Sharma V, et al. The use of thrombin injections in the management of bleeding gastric varices: a single center experience. Gastrointest Endosc 2008;68:877–82.
72. Yang WL, Tripathi D, Therapondos G, et al. Endoscopic use of human thrombin in bleeding gastric varices. Am J Gastroenterol 2002;97:1381–5.
73. Heneghan MA, Byrne A, Harrison PM. An open pilot study of the effects of a human fibrin glue for endoscopic treatment of patients with acute bleeding from gastric varices. Gastrointest Endosc 2002;56:422–6.
74. Datta D, Vlavianos P, Alisa A, et al. Use of fibrin glue (beriplast) in the management of bleeding gastric varices. Endoscopy 2003;35:675–8.
75. McAvoy NC, Hayes PC. The use of human thrombin for the treatment of gastric and ectopic varices. Gut 2006;55:A5.
76. Tripathi D, Hayes PC. Endoscopic therapy for bleeding gastric varices: to clot or glue? Gastrointest Endosc 2008;68:883–6.
77. Chun HJ, Hyun JH. A new method of endoscopic variceal ligation-injection sclerotherapy (EVLIS) for gastric varices. Korean J Intern Med 1995;10(2):108–19.
78. Takeuchi M, Nakai Y, Syu A, et al. Endoscopic ligation of gastric varices. Lancet 1996;348(9033):1038.
79. Miyazaki S, Yoshida T, Harada T, et al. Injection sclerotherapy for gastric varices using N-butyl-2-cyanoacrylate and ethanolamine oleate. Hepatogastroenterology 1998;45(22):1155–8.
80. Arakaki Y, Murakami K, Takahashi K, et al. Clinical evaluation of combined endoscopic variceal ligation and sclerotherapy of gastric varices in liver cirrhosis. Endoscopy 2003;35:940–5.
81. Sugimoto N, Watanabe K, Watanabe K, et al. Endoscopic hemostasis for bleeding gastric varices treated by combination of variceal ligation and sclerotherapy with N-butyl-2-cyanoacrylate. J Gastroenterol 2007;42:528–32.
82. Kuo MJ, Yeh HZ, Chen GH, et al. Improvement of tissue adhesive obliteration of bleeding gastric varices using adjuvant hypertonic glucose solution injection: a prospective randomized trial. Endoscopy 2007;39:487–91.
83. Chang KY, Wu CS, Chen PC. Endoscopic treatment of bleeding fundic varices with 50% glucose injection. Endoscopy 1996;28:398.
84. Yoshida T, Hayashi N, Suzumi N, et al. Endoscopic ligation of gastric varices using a detachable snare. Endoscopy 1994;26(5):502–5.

Management of Gastropathy and Gastric Vascular Ectasia in Portal Hypertension

Cristina Ripoll, MD[a], Guadalupe Garcia-Tsao, MD[b,*]

KEYWORDS

- Portal hypertensive gastropathy
- Gastric antral vascular ectasia • Portal hypertension
- Cirrhosis • Management

Patients with cirrhosis are at an increased risk of gastrointestinal hemorrhage, with the most common source being gastroesophageal varices. However, there are gastrointestinal mucosal lesions typical of cirrhosis that may also bleed in these patients, namely portal hypertensive gastropathy (PHG) and gastric antral vascular ectasia (GAVE). These are 2 clearly distinct mucosal lesions with different pathophysiology, endoscopic appearance, histopathology, and treatment (**Table 1**). PHG, as its name indicates, is associated with the presence of portal hypertension and therefore is only observed in patients with this condition, whereas GAVE is observed in patients without portal hypertension or liver disease. Nevertheless and despite the differences between both entities, they may lead to similar clinical manifestations, most frequently to symptoms caused by chronic ferropenic anemia associated with chronic occult blood loss, and only rarely lead to acute, overt gastrointestinal hemorrhage.

PHG

PHG is characterized by more or less typical gastric mucosal lesions presenting in patients with portal hypertension (either prehepatic or hepatic) (**Fig. 1**). Its typical location is in the gastric fundus and upper body of the stomach, although it can affect the

Supported by grants from the Centro de Investigación Biomédica en Red de Enfermedades Hepáticas y Digestivas (CIBERehd) and Yale Liver Center NIH P30 DK34989.
[a] Hepatology and Liver Transplant Unit, Department of Digestive Diseases, Area 6300, Hospital General Universitario Gregorio Marañón, Dr. Esquero 46, Madrid, Spain
[b] Section of Digestive Diseases, Yale University School of Medicine and VA-CT Healthcare System, 333 Cedar Street – 1080 LMP, New Haven, CT 06510, USA
* Corresponding author.
E-mail address: guadalupe.garcia-tsao@yale.edu

Clin Liver Dis 14 (2010) 281–295
doi:10.1016/j.cld.2010.03.013
1089-3261/10/$ – see front matter. Published by Elsevier Inc.

Table 1
Differential characteristics between PHG and GAVE

PHG		GAVE
Causal	Relationship with portal hypertension	Coincidental
Mainly proximal	Distribution in stomach	Mainly distal
+	Presence in other territories of GI tract	–
Mosaic pattern + red spots	Endoscopic findings	Linear pattern + red spots
Severe PHG	Difficult differential diagnosis	Diffuse GAVE
Dilated capillaries and venules No inflammation	Pathology	Thrombi Spindle cell proliferation Fibrohyalinosis
Portal pressure reducing	Treatment	Endoscopic
TIPS/shunt surgery	Salvage therapy[a]	Antrectomy and Billroth I

Abbreviations: GI, gastrointestinal; SMT, somatostatin.
[a] To be evaluated on an individual basis.

whole stomach and even other areas of the gastrointestinal tract, such as the small bowel or the colon.[1–8]

Epidemiology

The prevalence of PHG in patients with portal hypertension has been reported to vary between 20% and 80%.[1,9–12] The wide variation in the reported prevalence is most likely a result of differences in the study population, specifically the proportion of patients with noncirrhotic portal hypertension, the severity of the underlying liver disease, and the proportion of patients with previous endoscopic treatment. A higher rate of PHG is observed in patients with more severe liver disease[10,11] and in patients who have had previous endoscopic treatment with sclerotherapy or endoscopic variceal ligation.[1,9,12] There is controversy regarding the specific endoscopic technique

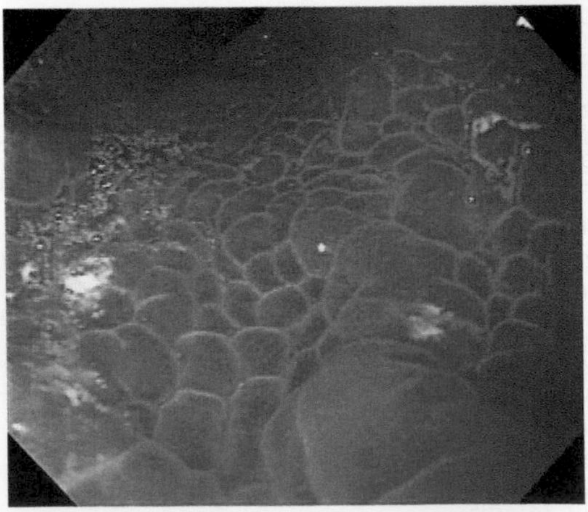

Fig. 1. Portal gastropathy with a snakeskin mosaic appearance in a cirrhotic patient who underwent an upper endoscopy for screening of varices.

used for variceal eradication that leads to a higher prevalence of PHG, with some studies showing a higher incidence after sclerotherapy than after ligation and other studies showing a similar incidence with both techniques.[13–15] Although many studies have concluded that the presence of PHG is associated with indirect signs of portal hypertension such as the presence of large varices,[1,11] splenomegaly,[10,11] and low platelet count,[11] the studies that evaluated the association between the hepatic venous pressure gradient (HVPG), a well-established method to measure portal pressure,[16] and PHG have led to controversial results. Two studies found no clear relationship between HVPG and PHG,[17,18] whereas another study found that patients with more severe gastropathy had a higher HVPG than patients with mild or no gastropathy.[19] These controversial results may be a result of selection bias, because all patients who were included in these studies had clinically significant portal hypertension.[17,18] The issue would be clearer if it could be shown that PHG presents only in patients with cirrhosis and portal hypertension (HVPG $\geq$ 6 mm Hg) or only in those with clinically significant portal hypertension (HVPG $\geq$ 10 mm Hg). However, such studies are still lacking.

Pathophysiology

The pathophysiology of PHG is unclear, although portal hypertension plays a major role. Studies that have evaluated the prevalence of PHG have revealed that it is almost exclusively observed in patients with portal hypertension, with or without liver disease.[20,21] PHG was not observed in 100 patients with chronic alcoholism without signs of liver disease or portal hypertension (on ultrasonographic examination) or in 10 patients with cirrhosis without portal hypertension.[21] It is not a peptic process, because mucosal changes do not respond to antisecretory drugs, and histologic changes, predominantly dilated capillaries and venules in the mucosa and submucosa without significant inflammation, are clearly distinct from those typically observed in peptic related disease.[22] Nevertheless, it seems that the gastric mucosa has an increased susceptibility to injury by noxious factors, as well as impaired healing.[23–26]

Diagnosis

The diagnosis of PHG, and by extension portal hypertensive enteropathy (similar mucosal changes at other sites of the gastrointestinal tract), is established when the characteristic endoscopic findings are observed in patients with portal hypertension. PHG is classified as mild when only the snakeskin mosaic pattern is present (see **Fig. 1**) or severe when, in addition to the mosaic pattern, flat or bulging red marks or black-brown spots are observed.[27] The clinical relevance of this classification has been established because patients with severe PHG are more likely to have acute bleeding or chronic anemia than patients with mild PHG.[11,28] Furthermore, this classification is reproducible as a good concordance between observers has been shown, especially regarding the mosaic pattern and red marks.[28] Similar lesions to the ones observed in the stomach in patients with PHG have been observed in the small bowel[3,5,7,29,30] and the colon.[2,7]

Some studies have evaluated alternative nonendoscopic methods for the diagnosis of PHG[31,32] such as magnetic resonance imaging or computed tomography, although until further evaluation in larger populations is available, endoscopy still remains the chief diagnostic method. In a study evaluating the efficacy of capsule endoscopy in the evaluation of the presence and size of varices, capsule endoscopy was shown to have only moderate sensitivity and specificity for the detection of PHG.[33] Future studies should specifically evaluate its efficacy in evaluating not only the presence but also the severity of PHG, as capsule endoscopy is particularly important in the evaluation of lesions in the small bowel.

Natural History

PHG may change with time in an individual patient. Studies that have evaluated the natural history of PHG have reported controversial results, possibly because of differences in study population. If only patients with cirrhosis who do not require primary or secondary prophylaxis are included, approximately 30% of patients with mild PHG develop severe PHG during a follow-up period ranging from 12 to 103 months.[11] Only a few cases of improvement in PHG have been reported. Most of the cases that bleed from PHG occur in patients with de novo PHG or in those with worsening of previous PHG.[9,11] Patients with diffuse lesions are more likely to bleed.[9,12] Patients who have PHG associated with cirrhosis-related portal hypertension have more frequently persistent and progressive PHG (which is more likely to bleed) than patients with PHG related to noncirrhotic portal hypertension.[9] Although, as mentioned earlier, patients with previous endoscopic therapy (sclerotherapy or endoscopic variceal ligation) have a higher prevalence of PHG,[1,9,12] the clinical course of the PHG in this setting, particularly in noncirrhotic portal hypertension, may be milder and transient.[9,14] Studies that have focused on patients with cirrhosis have not observed differences in severity or course of PHG in patients who develop it spontaneously or after endoscopic therapy.[1]

Clinical Picture

PHG is mostly asymptomatic but, when symptomatic, it most frequently causes chronic gastrointestinal blood loss and ferropenic anemia. No study has evaluated the prevalence of PHG in cirrhotic patients with chronic anemia. The rate of chronic hemorrhage in patients with PHG ranges between 6% and 60% in different studies.[1,9,11,34] This wide variation is a result of a great heterogeneity in the patient population included in the different studies, from patients without cirrhosis[9] to patients with cirrhosis and severe PHG.[34] Chronic bleeding from PHG is suspected in a patient with portal hypertension and chronic ferropenic anemia and its presence is confirmed on thorough examination of the whole gastrointestinal tract including upper endoscopy, colonoscopy, and evaluation of the small bowel, which is most easily achieved with capsule endoscopy.

Although PHG may bleed acutely, leading to hematemesis and/or melena, this accounts for only a few cases of acute gastrointestinal hemorrhage in patients with cirrhosis. In a study that included 250 patients with cirrhosis presenting with gastrointestinal hemorrhage in whom a source could be identified, PHG accounted for only 5% of the cases, with varices (57%) and peptic disease (17%) being the most frequent sources.[35] Studies that evaluate the probability of bleeding from PHG report an incidence between 2.5% and 30%,[1,9,11,34] with the greatest incidence observed in patients with severe PHG.[9,11,34] Diagnosis of acute hemorrhage from PHG is established when active bleeding from gastropathy lesions or nonremovable clots overlying these lesions is observed or when there is PHG and no other cause of acute bleeding can be noted after thorough evaluation of the gastrointestinal tract.

Management

Treatment of PHG relies on 2 main pillars (**Fig. 2**). First, general measures used in gastrointestinal bleeding independent of cause should be applied and second a specific approach to treat the cause of the gastrointestinal bleed should be undertaken. The most effective specific treatments in patients with PHG are those aimed at

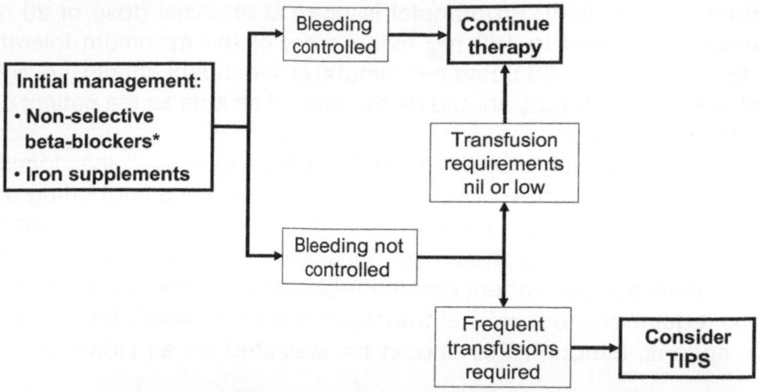

Fig. 2. Algorithm for the management of chronic bleeding from portal hypertensive gastropathy. *Adjusted to the maximal dose tolerated (goal is heart rate ~55 beats per minute); heart rate should be checked at each visit to ensure compliance.

reducing portal pressure. The main pharmacologic agent that has been investigated in this setting is the nonselective β-blocker propranolol.

Chronic hemorrhage

In the most frequent context of chronic blood loss, iron supplementation should be provided to counteract the continuous depletion of iron deposits. The most effective specific therapy is that aimed at reducing portal pressure. Nonselective β-blockers have been shown to decrease bleeding from acute and chronic forms of hemorrhage from PHG. The first trial[36] was a randomized controlled trial that included only 24 patients. Patients with portal hypertension shown by the presence of varices and PHG diagnosed at least 6 weeks before inclusion were randomized to the administration of long-acting propranolol (160 mg/d) or placebo initially for 6 weeks and then crossed over to the other arm for another 6 weeks. While patients were on propranolol, there was a lower rate of hemorrhage, an increase in hemoglobin level and an apparent improvement in the endoscopic appearance of the lesions, compared with the placebo period. However, the study was too underpowered to yield any significant statistical or clinical conclusions.

More solid evidence supporting the use of propranolol in the prevention of recurrent bleeding in patients with cirrhosis and severe PHG was obtained from a randomized controlled trial in which patients who had previously bled acutely or chronically from PHG were randomized to receive propranolol (26 patients) or no therapy other than iron administration if needed (28 patients).[34] The end point of the trial was recurrent hemorrhage from PHG. This criterion was defined as (1) the presence of acute upper gastrointestinal bleeding with a decrease in hematocrit and the finding on emergency endoscopy (performed within the first 12 hours) of gastric red spots as the source of bleeding, or (2) the presence of chronic bleeding defined by occult blood loss with transfusion requirements of 3 or more units of red packed blood cells in 3 months or continuous iron replacement therapy for more than 50% of the time of follow-up. The actuarial probability of remaining free of hemorrhage was greater in patients randomized to propranolol in the acute (85% vs 20%) and in the chronic setting (63% vs 40% at 30 months), although in the latter this difference did not achieve statistical significance.[34] On multivariate analysis, the only independent predictor of recurrent hemorrhage was the absence of propranolol.[34] Therefore, nonselective β-blockers should be used in the chronic setting and in the acute setting (once the acute episode is controlled). Propranolol is given at an initial dose of 20 mg twice a day, gradually escalated to 160 mg twice a day or the maximum tolerated dose according to heart rate (50–55 beats per minute) or secondary effects (eg, light-headedness, asthenia). This therapy should be maintained as long as the patient continues to have portal hypertension.

Use of other pharmacologic agents in PHG such as losartan,[37] thalidomide,[38] and corticosteroids[39] has been described. However, the evidence supporting the use of these agents is weak as they are based on small open-label studies and case reports.

Nonresponse to β-blockers should be considered when the patient continues to bleed and is transfusion dependent despite β-blockers and iron replacement therapy. Patients who require only occasional transfusions do not benefit from more invasive therapeutic options, although this should be evaluated on an individual basis (see **Fig. 2**).

Because portal hypertension is the main underlying factor that leads to the development of PHG, shunt therapies have been evaluated as salvage therapies. Data have been reported regarding the use of the transjugular intrahepatic portosystemic shunt (TIPS)[40–43] and shunt surgery.[44,45] TIPS placement consists of the creation of a shunt between a hepatic vein and a portal vein. From a hemodynamic point of view it is similar to a side-to-side surgical portacaval shunt and is effective in lowering portal pressure. Almost all patients who receive TIPS show an improvement of PHG lesions on endoscopic evaluation and a decrease in transfusion requirements.[40–43] In the largest study (40 patients with PHG) endoscopic improvement was detected as early as 6 weeks after TIPS placement, although in patients with severe PHG it could take at least 3 months.[40] Similar results have been shown with shunt surgery (ie, improvement in endoscopic appearance and lower transfusion requirements).[44,45] Because of the morbidity associated with shunt surgery, particularly in patients with cirrhosis, its role may be more relevant in patients with noncirrhotic portal hypertension.[45]

Only 1 study has evaluated the use of endoscopic treatment of PHG with argon plasma coagulation (APC).[46] This study included 29 patients, of whom 11 were considered to be bleeding from PHG, defined as diffuse vascular ectasia with a background mosaic pattern distributed throughout the stomach in patients with portal hypertension. The APC was set at 30 to 40 W and 1.5 to 2 L/min of argon plasma flow. The aim of each session was to ablate as much of the surface as possible (at least 80% of the mucosa in diffuse lesions). Sessions were repeated as needed every 2 to 4 weeks. The treatment success, defined by the absence of further episodes of upper gastrointestinal bleeding or a reduction in blood transfusion requirements, was between 81% and 90% without any significant differences between groups. The data are limited and this endoscopic approach could be considered in patients in whom severe recurrent bleeding occurs despite β-blockers and who are not candidates for TIPS.

Acute hemorrhage

Although PHG may present as acute gastrointestinal hemorrhage, this presentation is less frequent than chronic blood loss. As in all patients with acute hemorrhage, general measures should be undertaken. Adequate volume resuscitation should be provided. Even although data specific for acute hemorrhage from PHG are not available given its low frequency, it seems reasonable to apply general measures proven to be efficacious in improving outcomes in patients with acute variceal hemorrhage such as cautious blood transfusion aimed at maintaining a hemoglobin level of around 8 g/dL and the use of short-term prophylactic antibiotics.[47] Oral or intravenous quinolones are the recommended antibiotics such as norfloxacin (400 mg twice a day) or ciprofloxacin (500 mg twice a day by mouth or 200 mg twice a day intravenously). Intravenous ceftriaxone (1 g/d) may be preferred in patients with Child B or C cirrhosis, or in those undergoing prophylaxis with quinolones.[48]

Besides the general measures, a specific portal hypotensive approach should be undertaken. The use of β-blockers in the acute setting was evaluated in an open trial in acute severe bleeding from endoscopically proven PHG (14 patients).[36] In this context, all but 1 patient ceased to bleed within 3 days of the initiation of propranolol.[36] However, the gradual dose titration of the drug necessary to achieve adequate β-blockade is not ideal. Blunting the physiologic compensatory increase in heart rate that results from acute bleeding seems counterintuitive. In this setting, vasoactive drugs used routinely in the setting of variceal hemorrhage such as somatostatin and its analogues (octreotide and vapreotide) and vasopressin and its analogue terlipressin, which are effective by means of producing a decrease in portal pressure,[49,50] appear to be useful. Three trials have evaluated the use of these drugs in acute hemorrhage from PHG.[51–53] Hemorrhage was satisfactorily controlled with somatostatin,[53] octreotide,[52,53] or terlipressin,[51] although vasopressin[52] did not show any benefit compared with omeprazole. Furthermore, in the trial that evaluated the effect of terlipressin, patients who received a larger (1 mg/4 h) dose of terlipressin had a higher proportion of control of hemorrhage and a lower recurrence rate than those who received a lower dose (0.2 mg/4 h).[51]

Therefore, following current recommendations,[47] resuscitation, a safe vasoactive drug (somatostatin or terlipressin), and antibiotic prophylaxis should be started as soon as gastrointestinal bleeding is suspected in a patient with cirrhosis, preferably before upper endoscopy. It seems reasonable that once the diagnosis of bleeding caused by PHG is established, these drugs should be maintained.

In acute hemorrhage that does not respond to medical treatment, alternative approaches should be contemplated. Nonresponse to medical treatment in the acute setting may be defined according to the standards of nonresponse to variceal bleeding,[27] as both are associated with portal hypertension and require a change of therapy. Treatment failure is considered when there is a new hematemesis after at least 2 hours of treatment initiation, or a 3-g drop in hemoglobin in the absence of transfusion of packed red blood cells or an inadequate hemoglobin increase in response to blood transfusions, or death.[27]

Rescue therapies in patients in whom standard therapy fails are the same as those recommended in patients who fail standard therapy for chronic bleeding (see **Fig. 2**).

GAVE

GAVE is characterized by the presence of red spots without a background mosaic pattern that are typically located in the gastric antrum. GAVE is most frequently observed in patients with cirrhosis and portal hypertension, although it has also been observed in patients without cirrhosis such as those with autoimmune connective tissue disorders, bone marrow transplantation, or chronic renal failure.[54–57] Seemingly, patients with cirrhosis more often have diffuse disease[58] whereas in noncirrhotic patients the disease is most frequently limited to the antrum.[59,60] In contrast to PHG, GAVE is observed only in the stomach and not in other parts of the gastrointestinal tract.

The prevalence of GAVE in cirrhosis is low. In a recent study performed in patients awaiting liver transplantation, GAVE was observed in only 8 of 345 (2%) of the patients.[61] A similar prevalence has been described in patients with the hepatitis C virus and advanced fibrosis.[10]

Pathophysiology

The pathophysiology of GAVE is not fully understood. In patients with cirrhosis, portal hypertension seems not to be essential in its development because patients do not respond to portal pressure-reducing therapies, such as TIPS or surgical shunt.[40,62] Liver insufficiency seems to play a significant role in the development of GAVE because it develops in patients with more severe liver dysfunction[59] and it has been shown to resolve after liver transplantation.[61,63] Speculation regarding an accumulation of substances not metabolized by the liver that may induce vasodilatation and/or angiogenesis has been suggested as a possible mechanism.[62] The association between GAVE and hormones with vasodilating properties such as gastrin[18,54,59] and prostaglandin E_2[64] has also been suggested. Abnormal antral motility[65] and mechanical stress[18] have also been associated with the pathogenesis of GAVE, which is further supported by the antral distribution of the lesions.

Diagnosis

The diagnosis of GAVE is established when the characteristic red spots (without a background mosaic pattern) are seen in the stomach at endoscopy. These lesions are typically found in the antrum, and are sometimes aggregated in a linear distribution, so that one may observe red longitudinal stripes that may be flat or raised, with visible blood vessels and pale normal mucosa in between, similar to a watermelon, hence the term watermelon stomach.[54] The lesions may be distributed diffusely throughout the proximal and distal stomach. In these cases the term diffuse GAVE is preferred.[54] The appearance of diffuse GAVE may be similar to severe PHG and it is important to differentiate them because treatment is different.[66]

istologically, GAVE lesions are completely distinct from PHG. Therefore, biopsy can be used to distinguish between these 2 entities, particularly in those cases in which the endoscopic appearance of the lesions may lead to some confusion (**Table 1**).[59] Findings in full-thickness mucosal biopsies that are highly suggestive of GAVE are mucosal vascular ectasia, fibrin thombi, fibrohyalinosis, and spindle cell proliferation without signs of inflammation. However, the absence of these characteristics on biopsy does not preclude the diagnosis of GAVE because biopsies are normally not deep enough.[67]

Clinical Presentation

From a clinical perspective, GAVE presents in a similar manner to PHG, that is, although most patients are completely asymptomatic, others present with acute or chronic hemorrhage and iron deficiency anemia. Acute hemorrhage seems to be more frequent in patients with cirrhosis, whereas noncirrhotic patients generally present with anemia.[60] In a study in which patients (with or without cirrhosis) underwent endoscopic evaluation of nonvariceal upper gastrointestinal hemorrhage, GAVE was the cause of hemorrhage in 26 of 744 patients (4%). Approximately one-third of these patients with GAVE had underlying portal hypertension.[58]

Management

In the setting of acute hemorrhage, the general therapeutic measures recommended for patients with cirrhosis and acute hemorrhage from varices or PHG (see earlier discussion) apply to patients with cirrhosis who bleed acutely from GAVE.

Specific measures to treat patients with GAVE with acute or chronic bleeding are substantially different from those used in PHG (**Fig. 3**). The mainstay of therapy in GAVE is the endoscopic ablation of the lesions (see **Fig. 3**). Some other studies

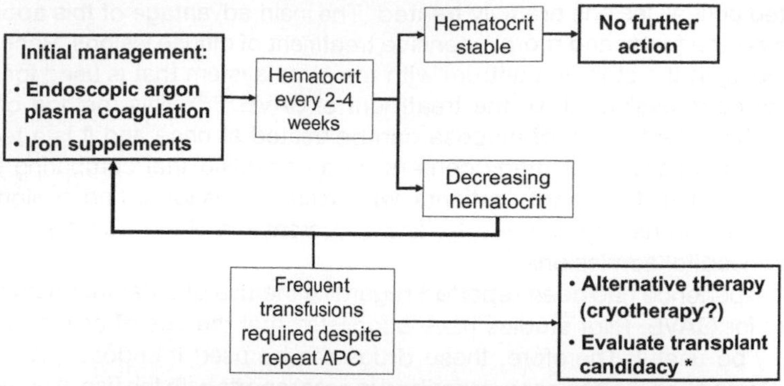

Fig. 3. Algorithm for the management of chronic bleeding from gastric antral vascular ectasia. *Because GAVE has been reported to resolve after liver transplant, in a patient who otherwise meets criteria for liver transplant, evaluation should be expedited.

have evaluated the use of different drugs and other more invasive options, but these should be used once endoscopic therapy has failed.

Many different endoscopic approaches have been used in the setting of GAVE although most studies have evaluated the use of thermoablative techniques. Typically several sessions are needed to achieve a control of acute bleeding and to correct anemia caused by chronic blood loss.

The most numerous studies evaluating the use of thermoablative methods in the treatment of GAVE are with APC, which produces thermal coagulation by applying high-frequency electric current that is passed through with argon gas without direct contact with the mucosa. Several studies have reported the beneficial effect of this method in patients with GAVE.[46,58,60,68–74] The main advantage of APC is that it is easy to use and the risk of perforation is lower than with Nd:YAG laser. Large areas of mucosa may be treated in a single session, although this is time consuming. Complications associated with this method are the development of hyperplasic polyps[74–76] and gastric outlet obstruction.[73,77] The settings for the electrical power (20–80 W) and gas flow (0.5–2 L/min) vary throughout the studies. The technique combines focal pulse and paintbrush. The sessions should be repeated every 2 to 6 weeks as needed.

The use of neodymium:yttrium-aluminum-garnet (Nd:YAG) laser coagulation has also shown to be effective in reducing rebleeding and transfusion requirements.[54,56,78–81] Its main advantage is that it can be applied to a large surface area of the mucosa in a single session and that its hemostatic response may be observed earlier. On the other hand, the risk of perforation is greater than with other thermoablative approaches such as APC, because the thermal effect penetrates deeper. The Nd:YAG laser is placed 1 cm from the mucosa surface and is used with a power setting between 40 and 90 W with short pulse durations (0.5–1 seconds). Sessions should be repeated every 2 to 4 weeks until the therapeutic goal is achieved.

Other endoscopic therapeutic options such as sclerotherapy and heater probe ablation[82] do not seem to have significant advantages compared with the previously described methods. However, there are other endoscopic approaches with more limited experience that may offer some additional advantages. Cryotherapy[83,84] consists of rapid expansion in the stomach of compressed nitrous oxide, resulting in a local decrease of the temperature with consequent freezing of the mucosa. The cryospray is applied with a specific catheter until ice is formed. Endoscopy should be repeated until all lesions are fully treated. The main advantage of this approach is that it allows for a faster and more extensive treatment of diffuse lesions. Recently, the use of banding in the stomach antrum with the same system that is used for variceal ligation has been evaluated for the treatment of GAVE.[85,86] This method offers the advantage that a large area of mucosa can be treated at once and it is a technique that is easily accessible for many centers. In a controlled trial comparing banding with thermoablative treatment, patients who received banding had a significantly greater increase in hemoglobin levels, and a decrease in blood transfusion requirements and hospital admissions.[85]

Limited experience has been reported regarding the use of different pharmacologic treatments for GAVE. Pilot studies have suggested that the use of estrogen-progesterone may be useful. Therefore, these drugs can be used if endoscopic treatment fails.[87–89] Some success has been described in case reports with the use of octreotide,[90] corticosteroids,[91,92] tranexamic acid,[93] thalidomide,[94] and a serotonin antagonist.[95] Some cases have resolved with treatment of the underlying disease such as liver transplantation in patients with cirrhosis,[61,63] although there has been a report of worsening GAVE despite adequate control of the underlying disease (systemic sclerosis and interstitial pneumonitis).[96]

In extreme cases in which the combination of endoscopic and pharmacologic treatment is unsuccessful, surgery with antrectomy can be considered on an individual basis.[97–99] The preferred procedure is antrectomy with Billroth I anastomosis. A thorough endoscopic evaluation of the gastrointestinal tract should be performed to exclude other causes of bleeding before turning to surgery. This is the most definitive therapy, with low rates of rebleeding and anemia. However, morbidity and mortality are high, particularly in patients with decompensated cirrhosis in whom GAVE usually presents.

SUMMARY

PHG and GAVE are 2 different clinical entities that share a common clinical manifestation: gastrointestinal bleeding. Most cases present as chronic bleeding, although there may be some cases of acute life-threatening bleed. Besides the common clinical manifestation, these 2 entities are clearly distinct, with different pathophysiology, endoscopic appearance, and therapeutic approach. The treatment of PHG is based on measures that reduce portal pressure, namely the administration of β-blockers. On the other hand, GAVE responds to endoscopic treatment. Most studies in this context have used thermoablative techniques, mainly APC. Refractory cases can respond to more invasive therapeutic options, although this has to be evaluated on a case-by-case basis.

REFERENCES

1. Primignani M, Carpinelli L, Preatoni P, et al. Natural history of portal hypertensive gastropathy in patients with liver cirrhosis. The New Italian Endoscopic Club for the study and treatment of esophageal varices (NIEC). Gastroenterology 2000; 119(1):181–7.
2. Bresci G, Parisi G, Capria A. Clinical relevance of colonic lesions in cirrhotic patients with portal hypertension. Endoscopy 2006;38(8):830–5.
3. Figueiredo P, Almeida N, Lerias C, et al. Effect of portal hypertension in the small bowel: an endoscopic approach. Dig Dis Sci 2008;53(8):2144–50.
4. Goulas S, Triantafyllidou K, Karagiannis S, et al. Capsule endoscopy in the investigation of patients with portal hypertension and anemia. Can J Gastroenterol 2008;22(5):469–74.

5. Higaki N, Matsui H, Imaoka H, et al. Characteristic endoscopic features of portal hypertensive enteropathy. J Gastroenterol 2008;43(5):327–31.
6. Ito K, Shiraki K, Sakai T, et al. Portal hypertensive colopathy in patients with liver cirrhosis. World J Gastroenterol 2005;11(20):3127–30.
7. Menchen L, Ripoll C, Marin-Jimenez I, et al. Prevalence of portal hypertensive duodenopathy in cirrhosis: clinical and haemodynamic features. Eur J Gastroenterol Hepatol 2006;18(6):649–53.
8. Misra SP, Dwivedi M, Misra V. Prevalence and factors influencing hemorrhoids, anorectal varices, and colopathy in patients with portal hypertension. Endoscopy 1996;28(4):340–5.
9. Sarin SK, Shahi HM, Jain M, et al. The natural history of portal hypertensive gastropathy: influence of variceal eradication. Am J Gastroenterol 2000;95(10): 2888–93.
10. Fontana RJ, Sanyal AJ, Mehta S, et al. Portal hypertensive gastropathy in chronic hepatitis C patients with bridging fibrosis and compensated cirrhosis: results from the HALT-C trial. Am J Gastroenterol 2006;101(5):983–92.
11. Merli M, Nicolini G, Angeloni S, et al. The natural history of portal hypertensive gastropathy in patients with liver cirrhosis and mild portal hypertension. Am J Gastroenterol 2004;99(10):1959–65.
12. D'Amico G, Montalbano L, Traina M, et al. Natural history of congestive gastropathy in cirrhosis. The Liver Study Group of V. Cervello Hospital. Gastroenterology 1990;99(6):1558–64.
13. Yuksel O, Koklu S, Arhan M, et al. Effects of esophageal varice eradication on portal hypertensive gastropathy and fundal varices: a retrospective and comparative study. Dig Dis Sci 2006;51(1):27–30.
14. Hou MC, Lin HC, Chen CH, et al. Changes in portal hypertensive gastropathy after endoscopic variceal sclerotherapy or ligation: an endoscopic observation. Gastrointest Endosc 1995;42(2):139–44.
15. Yoshikawa I, Murata I, Nakano S, et al. Effects of endoscopic variceal ligation on portal hypertensive gastropathy and gastric mucosal blood flow. Am J Gastroenterol 1998;93(1):71–4.
16. Groszmann RJ, Wongcharatrawee S. The hepatic venous pressure gradient: anything worth doing should be done right. Hepatology 2004;39(2):280–2.
17. Bellis L, Nicodemo S, Galossi A, et al. Hepatic venous pressure gradient does not correlate with the presence and the severity of portal hypertensive gastropathy in patients with liver cirrhosis. J Gastrointestin Liver Dis 2007;16(3):273–7.
18. Quintero E, Pique JM, Bombi JA, et al. Gastric mucosal vascular ectasias causing bleeding in cirrhosis. A distinct entity associated with hypergastrinemia and low serum levels of pepsinogen I. Gastroenterology 1987;93(5):1054–61.
19. Iwao T, Toyonaga A, Sumino M, et al. Portal hypertensive gastropathy in patients with cirrhosis. Gastroenterology 1992;102(6):2060–5.
20. Sarin SK, Misra SP, Singal A, et al. Evaluation of the incidence and significance of the "mosaic pattern" in patients with cirrhosis, noncirrhotic portal fibrosis, and extrahepatic obstruction. Am J Gastroenterol 1988;83(11):1235–9.
21. Papazian A, Braillon A, Dupas JL, et al. Portal hypertensive gastric mucosa: an endoscopic study. Gut 1986;27(10):1199–203.
22. McCormack TT, Sims J, Eyre-Brook I, et al. Gastric lesions in portal hypertension: inflammatory gastritis or congestive gastropathy? Gut 1985;26(11):1226–32.
23. Kawanaka H, Tomikawa M, Jones MK, et al. Defective mitogen-activated protein kinase (ERK2) signaling in gastric mucosa of portal hypertensive rats: potential therapeutic implications. Hepatology 2001;34(5):990–9.

24. Kinjo N, Kawanaka H, Akahoshi T, et al. Significance of ERK nitration in portal hypertensive gastropathy and its therapeutic implications. Am J Physiol Gastrointest Liver Physiol 2008;295(5):G1016–24.
25. Sarfeh IJ, Soliman H, Waxman K, et al. Impaired oxygenation of gastric mucosa in portal hypertension. The basis for increased susceptibility to injury. Dig Dis Sci 1989;34(2):225–8.
26. Sarfeh IJ, Tarnawski A. Gastric mucosal vasculopathy in portal hypertension. Gastroenterology 1987;93(5):1129–31.
27. de Franchis R. Evolving consensus in portal hypertension. Report of the Baveno IV consensus workshop on methodology of diagnosis and therapy in portal hypertension. J Hepatol 2005;43(1):167–76.
28. Stewart CA, Sanyal AJ. Grading portal gastropathy: validation of a gastropathy scoring system. Am J Gastroenterol 2003;98(8):1758–65.
29. Canlas KR, Dobozi BM, Lin S, et al. Using capsule endoscopy to identify GI tract lesions in cirrhotic patients with portal hypertension and chronic anemia. J Clin Gastroenterol 2008;42(7):844–8.
30. Barakat M, Mostafa M, Mahran Z, et al. Portal hypertensive duodenopathy: clinical, endoscopic, and histopathologic profiles. Am J Gastroenterol 2007;102(12):2793–802.
31. Erden A, Idilman R, Erden I, et al. Veins around the esophagus and the stomach: do their calibrations provide a diagnostic clue for portal hypertensive gastropathy? Clin Imaging 2009;33(1):22–4.
32. Ishihara K, Ishida R, Saito T, et al. Computed tomography features of portal hypertensive gastropathy. J Comput Assist Tomogr 2004;28(6):832–5.
33. de Franchis R, Eisen GM, Laine L, et al. Esophageal capsule endoscopy for screening and surveillance of esophageal varices in patients with portal hypertension. Hepatology 2008;47(5):1595–603.
34. Perez-Ayuso RM, Pique JM, Bosch J, et al. Propranolol in prevention of recurrent bleeding from severe portal hypertensive gastropathy in cirrhosis. Lancet 1991; 337(8755):1431–4.
35. Gostout CJ, Viggiano TR, Balm RK. Acute gastrointestinal bleeding from portal hypertensive gastropathy: prevalence and clinical features. Am J Gastroenterol 1993;88(12):2030–3.
36. Hosking SW. Congestive gastropathy in portal hypertension: variations in prevalence. Hepatology 1989;10(2):257–8.
37. Wagatsuma Y, Naritaka Y, Shimakawa T, et al. Clinical usefulness of the angiotensin II receptor antagonist losartan in patients with portal hypertensive gastropathy. Hepatogastroenterology 2006;53(68):171–4.
38. Karajeh MA, Hurlstone DP, Stephenson TJ, et al. Refractory bleeding from portal hypertensive gastropathy: a further novel role for thalidomide therapy? Eur J Gastroenterol Hepatol 2006;18(5):545–8.
39. Cremers MI, Oliveira AP, Alves AL, et al. Portal hypertensive gastropathy: treatment with corticosteroids. Endoscopy 2002;34(2):177.
40. Kamath PS, Lacerda M, Ahlquist DA, et al. Gastric mucosal responses to intrahepatic portosystemic shunting in patients with cirrhosis. Gastroenterology 2000; 118(5):905–11.
41. Mezawa S, Homma H, Ohta H, et al. Effect of transjugular intrahepatic portosystemic shunt formation on portal hypertensive gastropathy and gastric circulation. Am J Gastroenterol 2001;96(4):1155–9.
42. Urata J, Yamashita Y, Tsuchigame T, et al. The effects of transjugular intrahepatic portosystemic shunt on portal hypertensive gastropathy. J Gastroenterol Hepatol 1998;13(10):1061–7.

43. Vignali C, Bargellini I, Grosso M, et al. TIPS with expanded polytetrafluoroethylene-covered stent: results of an Italian multicenter study. AJR Am J Roentgenol 2005;185(2):472–80.
44. Orloff MJ, Orloff MS, Orloff SL, et al. Treatment of bleeding from portal hypertensive gastropathy by portacaval shunt. Hepatology 1995;21(4):1011–7.
45. Soin AS, Acharya SK, Mathur M, et al. Portal hypertensive gastropathy in noncirrhotic patients. The effect of lienorenal shunts. J Clin Gastroenterol 1998;26(1): 64–7 [discussion: 68].
46. Herrera S, Bordas JM, Llach J, et al. The beneficial effects of argon plasma coagulation in the management of different types of gastric vascular ectasia lesions in patients admitted for GI hemorrhage. Gastrointest Endosc 2008;68(3):440–6.
47. Garcia-Tsao G, Sanyal AJ, Grace ND, et al. Prevention and management of gastroesophageal varices and variceal hemorrhage in cirrhosis. Hepatology 2007;46(3):922–38.
48. Fernandez J, Ruiz del Arbol L, Gomez C, et al. Norfloxacin vs ceftriaxone in the prophylaxis of infections in patients with advanced cirrhosis and hemorrhage. Gastroenterology 2006;131(4):1049–56. [quiz: 1285].
49. Villanueva C, Planella M, Aracil C, et al. Hemodynamic effects of terlipressin and high somatostatin dose during acute variceal bleeding in nonresponders to the usual somatostatin dose. Am J Gastroenterol 2005;100(3):624–30.
50. Cirera I, Feu F, Luca A, et al. Effects of bolus injections and continuous infusions of somatostatin and placebo in patients with cirrhosis: a double-blind hemodynamic investigation. Hepatology 1995;22(1):106–11.
51. Bruha R, Marecek Z, Spicak J, et al. Double-blind randomized, comparative multicenter study of the effect of terlipressin in the treatment of acute esophageal variceal and/or hypertensive gastropathy bleeding. Hepatogastroenterology 2002;49(46):1161–6.
52. Zhou Y, Qiao L, Wu J, et al. Comparison of the efficacy of octreotide, vasopressin, and omeprazole in the control of acute bleeding in patients with portal hypertensive gastropathy: a controlled study. J Gastroenterol Hepatol 2002;17(9):973–9.
53. Kouroumalis EA, Koutroubakis IE, Manousos ON. Somatostatin for acute severe bleeding from portal hypertensive gastropathy. Eur J Gastroenterol Hepatol 1998; 10(6):509–12.
54. Gostout CJ, Viggiano TR, Ahlquist DA, et al. The clinical and endoscopic spectrum of the watermelon stomach. J Clin Gastroenterol 1992;15(3):256–63.
55. Tobin RW, Hackman RC, Kimmey MB, et al. Bleeding from gastric antral vascular ectasia in marrow transplant patients. Gastrointest Endosc 1996;44(3):223–9.
56. Liberski SM, McGarrity TJ, Hartle RJ, et al. The watermelon stomach: long-term outcome in patients treated with Nd:YAG laser therapy. Gastrointest Endosc 1994;40(5):584–7.
57. Yamamoto M, Takahashi H, Akaike J, et al. Gastric antral vascular ectasia (GAVE) associated with systemic sclerosis. Scand J Rheumatol 2008;37(4):315–6.
58. Dulai GS, Jensen DM, Kovacs TO, et al. Endoscopic treatment outcomes in watermelon stomach patients with and without portal hypertension. Endoscopy 2004;36(1):68–72.
59. Payen JL, Cales P, Voigt JJ, et al. Severe portal hypertensive gastropathy and antral vascular ectasia are distinct entities in patients with cirrhosis. Gastroenterology 1995;108(1):138–44.
60. Lecleire S, Ben-Soussan E, Antonietti M, et al. Bleeding gastric vascular ectasia treated by argon plasma coagulation: a comparison between patients with and without cirrhosis. Gastrointest Endosc 2008;67(2):219–25.

61. Ward EM, Raimondo M, Rosser BG, et al. Prevalence and natural history of gastric antral vascular ectasia in patients undergoing orthotopic liver transplantation. J Clin Gastroenterol 2004;38(10):898–900.
62. Spahr L, Villeneuve JP, Dufresne MP, et al. Gastric antral vascular ectasia in cirrhotic patients: absence of relation with portal hypertension. Gut 1999;44(5):739–42.
63. Vincent C, Pomier-Layrargues G, Dagenais M, et al. Cure of gastric antral vascular ectasia by liver transplantation despite persistent portal hypertension: a clue for pathogenesis. Liver Transpl 2002;8(8):717–20.
64. Saperas E, Perez Ayuso RM, Poca E, et al. Increased gastric PGE2 biosynthesis in cirrhotic patients with gastric vascular ectasia. Am J Gastroenterol 1990;85(2):138–44.
65. Charneau J, Petit R, Cales P, et al. Antral motility in patients with cirrhosis with or without gastric antral vascular ectasia. Gut 1995;37(4):488–92.
66. Burak KW, Lee SS, Beck PL. Portal hypertensive gastropathy and gastric antral vascular ectasia (GAVE) syndrome. Gut 2001;49(6):866–72.
67. Suit PF, Petras RE, Bauer TW, et al. Gastric antral vascular ectasia. A histologic and morphometric study of "the watermelon stomach". Am J Surg Pathol 1987;11(10):750–7.
68. Sato T, Yamazaki K, Toyota J, et al. Efficacy of argon plasma coagulation for gastric antral vascular ectasia associated with chronic liver disease. Hepatol Res 2005;32(2):121–6.
69. Yusoff I, Brennan F, Ormonde D, et al. Argon plasma coagulation for treatment of watermelon stomach. Endoscopy 2002;34(5):407–10.
70. Sebastian S, McLoughlin R, Qasim A, et al. Endoscopic argon plasma coagulation for the treatment of gastric antral vascular ectasia (watermelon stomach): long-term results. Dig Liver Dis 2004;36(3):212–7.
71. Roman S, Saurin JC, Dumortier J, et al. Tolerance and efficacy of argon plasma coagulation for controlling bleeding in patients with typical and atypical manifestations of watermelon stomach. Endoscopy 2003;35(12):1024–8.
72. Kwan V, Bourke MJ, Williams SJ, et al. Argon plasma coagulation in the management of symptomatic gastrointestinal vascular lesions: experience in 100 consecutive patients with long-term follow-up. Am J Gastroenterol 2006;101(1):58–63.
73. Probst A, Scheubel R, Wienbeck M. Treatment of watermelon stomach (GAVE syndrome) by means of endoscopic argon plasma coagulation (APC): long-term outcome. Z Gastroenterol 2001;39(6):447–52.
74. Fuccio L, Zagari RM, Serrani M, et al. Endoscopic argon plasma coagulation for the treatment of gastric antral vascular ectasia-related bleeding in patients with liver cirrhosis. Digestion 2009;79(3):143–50.
75. Baudet JS, Salata H, Soler M, et al. Hyperplastic gastric polyps after argon plasma coagulation treatment of gastric antral vascular ectasia (GAVE). Endoscopy 2007;39(Suppl 1):E320.
76. Izquierdo S, Rey E, Gutierrez Del Olmo A, et al. Polyp as a complication of argon plasma coagulation in watermelon stomach. Endoscopy 2005;37(9):921.
77. Farooq FT, Wong RC, Yang P, et al. Gastric outlet obstruction as a complication of argon plasma coagulation for watermelon stomach. Gastrointest Endosc 2007;65(7):1090–2.
78. Labenz J, Borsch G. Bleeding watermelon stomach treated by Nd-YAG laser photocoagulation. Endoscopy 1993;25(3):240–2.

79. Mathou NG, Lovat LB, Thorpe SM, et al. Nd:YAG laser induces long-term remission in transfusion-dependent patients with watermelon stomach. Lasers Med Sci 2004;18(4):213–8.
80. Selinger RR, McDonald GB, Hockenbery DM, et al. Efficacy of neodymium:YAG laser therapy for gastric antral vascular ectasia (GAVE) following hematopoietic cell transplant. Bone Marrow Transplant 2006;37(2):191–7.
81. Ng I, Lai KC, Ng M. Clinical and histological features of gastric antral vascular ectasia: successful treatment with endoscopic laser therapy. J Gastroenterol Hepatol 1996;11(3):270–4.
82. Petrini JL Jr, Johnston JH. Heat probe treatment for antral vascular ectasia. Gastrointest Endosc 1989;35(4):324–8.
83. Kantsevoy SV, Cruz-Correa MR, Vaughn CA, et al. Endoscopic cryotherapy for the treatment of bleeding mucosal vascular lesions of the GI tract: a pilot study. Gastrointest Endosc 2003;57(3):403–6.
84. Cho S, Zanati S, Yong E, et al. Endoscopic cryotherapy for the management of gastric antral vascular ectasia. Gastrointest Endosc 2008;68(5):895–902.
85. Wells CD, Harrison ME, Gurudu SR, et al. Treatment of gastric antral vascular ectasia (watermelon stomach) with endoscopic band ligation. Gastrointest Endosc 2008;68(2):231–6.
86. Gill KR, Raimondo M, Wallace MB. Endoscopic band ligation for the treatment of gastric antral vascular ectasia. Gastrointest Endosc 2009;69(6):1194.
87. Tran A, Villeneuve JP, Bilodeau M, et al. Treatment of chronic bleeding from gastric antral vascular ectasia (GAVE) with estrogen-progesterone in cirrhotic patients: an open pilot study. Am J Gastroenterol 1999;94(10):2909–11.
88. Manning RJ. Estrogen/progesterone treatment of diffuse antral vascular ectasia. Am J Gastroenterol 1995;90(1):154–6.
89. Moss SF, Ghosh P, Thomas DM, et al. Gastric antral vascular ectasia: maintenance treatment with oestrogen-progesterone. Gut 1992;33(5):715–7.
90. Nardone G, Rocco A, Balzano T, et al. The efficacy of octreotide therapy in chronic bleeding due to vascular abnormalities of the gastrointestinal tract. Aliment Pharmacol Ther 1999;13(11):1429–36.
91. Bhowmick BK. Watermelon stomach treated with oral corticosteroid. J R Soc Med 1993;86(1):52.
92. Suzuki T, Hirano M, Oka H. Long-term corticosteroid therapy for gastric antral vascular ectasia. Am J Gastroenterol 1996;91(9):1873–4.
93. McCormick PA, Ooi H, Crosbie O. Tranexamic acid for severe bleeding gastric antral vascular ectasia in cirrhosis. Gut 1998;42(5):750–2.
94. Dunne KA, Hill J, Dillon JF. Treatment of chronic transfusion-dependent gastric antral vascular ectasia (watermelon stomach) with thalidomide. Eur J Gastroenterol Hepatol 2006;18(4):455–6.
95. Cabral JE, Pontes JM, Toste M, et al. Watermelon stomach: treatment with a serotonin antagonist. Am J Gastroenterol 1991;86(7):927–8.
96. Shibukawa G, Irisawa A, Sakamoto N, et al. Gastric antral vascular ectasia (GAVE) associated with systemic sclerosis: relapse after endoscopic treatment by argon plasma coagulation. Intern Med 2007;46(6):279–83.
97. Mann NS, Rachut E. Gastric antral vascular ectasia causing severe hypoalbuminemia and anemia cured by antrectomy. J Clin Gastroenterol 2002;34(3):284–6.
98. Pljesa S, Golubovic G, Tomasevic R, et al. "Watermelon stomach" in patients on chronic hemodialysis. Ren Fail 2005;27(5):643–6.
99. Jabbari M, Cherry R, Lough JO, et al. Gastric antral vascular ectasia: the watermelon stomach. Gastroenterology 1984;87(5):1165–70.

Refractory Acute Variceal Bleeding: What to Do Next?

Mario D'Amico, MD[a], Annalisa Berzigotti, MD, PhD[a,b],
Juan Carlos Garcia-Pagan, MD, PhD[a,*]

KEYWORDS

- Portal hypertension • TIPS • Acute variceal bleeding
- Treatment failure

Variceal bleeding is a severe complication of portal hypertension, causing 70% of all upper gastrointestinal bleeding episodes in patients with liver cirrhosis.[1]

Data from placebo-controlled clinical trials show that variceal bleeding is spontaneously controlled in 40% to 50% of patients.[2] Standardization in supportive and new therapeutic treatments has reduced the bleeding-related mortality within the last 30 years from about 50% to 15% to 20%.[1] Current recommendations[3,4] for the treatment of acute variceal bleeding (AVB) are to combine hemodynamic stabilization, antibiotic prophylaxis, pharmacologic agents such as terlipressin, somatostatin, or its analogues, and endoscopic treatment (**Fig. 1**). The general management of patients bleeding from varices is aimed at correcting hypovolemic shock with careful volume replacement and transfusion, and at preventing complications, such as bacterial infections, hepatic decompensation, or renal failure, which can occur independently of the cause of the hemorrhage. Vasoactive drug therapy must be started early (ideally during transfer to the hospital, even if active bleeding is only suspected). Endoscopic band ligation (EBL) (or injection sclerotherapy if band ligation is technically difficult) must be performed after initial resuscitation when the patient is stable. However, despite the application of the current gold-standard pharmacologic and endoscopic

Grant support: Dr Mario D'Amico has received financial support from the Institut D'Investigacions Biomediques August Pi i Sunyer (IDIBAPS). This work was supported in part by grants from the Ministerio de Educaciòn y Ciencia (SAF 2007-61298). CIBERehd is funded by Instituto de Salud Carlos III.

[a] Hepatic Hemodynamic Laboratory, Liver Unit, Hospital Clinic, Institut d'Investigacions Biomediques August Pi i Sunyer (IDIBAPS) and Centro de Investigación Biomédica en Red de Enfermedades Hepáticas y Digestivas (CIBERehd), University of Barcelona, c/Villarroel 170, Barcelona 08036, Spain

[b] Ultrasound Unit, Centre de Diagnostic por la Imatge (CDIC), Hospital Clinic, University of Barcelona, c/Villarroel 170, Barcelona 08036, Spain

* Corresponding author.

E-mail address: jcgarcia@clinic.ub.es

Clin Liver Dis 14 (2010) 297–305
doi:10.1016/j.cld.2010.03.012
liver.theclinics.com

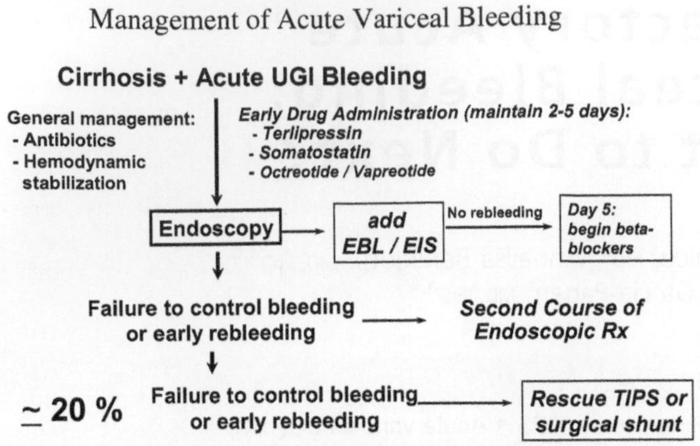

Fig. 1. The current recommendation for the treatment of AVB.

treatment, failure to control bleeding or early rebleed within 5 days still occurs in 15% to 20% of patients with AVB.[5] The mortality in these patients is high, approximately 30% to 50% in different series.[5,6] About 90% of deaths related to AVB are observed in this subgroup of patients, suggesting that failure of the initial treatment identifies patients at the highest risk of death.

This article reviews available therapies for treatment failures, and discusses strategies that can be applied to improve the outcome of these patients.

RESCUE THERAPIES FOR TREATMENT FAILURES

Definition of Treatment Failure

According to consensus,[3] treatment failure is defined as failure to control AVB within 24 hours, or failure to prevent clinically significant rebleeding or death within 5 days after treatment initiation. Failure to control bleeding within 24 hours or early rebleeding implies the need to change therapy.

Most of the data available regarding rescue therapies for refractory bleeding include a mixed population of patients, including those with treatment failure for the acute bleeding episode as well as patients with failure of the secondary prophylaxis to prevent rebleeding. The mixture of these 2 populations of patients, which are likely to have different outcomes regardless of the treatment used, may mask possible advantages or disadvantages of the different rescue treatments.

In case of treatment failure of the acute bleeding episode, if bleeding is mild and the patient is hemodynamically stable, a second endoscopic therapy may be attempted. If this fails, or if bleeding is severe, it is usually controlled temporarily with balloon tamponade until a definitive derivative treatment is applied.

Balloon Tamponade

Balloon tamponade is aimed at obtaining a temporary hemostasis by direct compression of bleeding varices. In experienced hands, balloon tamponade is highly successful in stopping bleeding,[7–11] but recurrence is observed in about half of the patients within 24 hours following deflation of the balloon. Major complications, the most lethal of which is esophageal rupture, have been observed in 6% to 20% of patients,[12] occurring more frequently in series in which tubes were inserted by inexperienced staff.[7] Therefore, tamponade should only be used by skilled and experienced staff.

The tubes should be used cautiously in patients with respiratory failure, cardiac arrhythmias, or hiatal hernia.

Preliminary studies[13–15] evaluated the use of self-expandable esophageal metallic stents as an alternative treatment to balloon tamponade for the temporary control of bleeding in treatment failures. In these studies stents had a high success rate with minor complications. However, before the extension of the use of this esophageal stents, these preliminary data must be confirmed in adequately designed trials.

The methods mentioned earlier are temporary and therefore once the patient is stabilized, a more definitive therapy such as surgery or a transjugular intrahepatic portosystemic shunt (TIPS) should be instituted.

Surgery

There are 2 basic types of operations: those that derive blood flow from the portal venous axis (shunt operations) and those that do not (nonshunt operations). Shunt operations can be categorized as nonselective (if they derive all portal blood flow to the inferior vena cava bypassing the liver, such as portacaval shunt [PCS]), and selective (if they are intended to at least partly preserve the portal blood flow to the liver, such as the distal splenorenal shunt [DSRS] or the calibrated small-diameter portacaval H-graft shunt). However, it is now accepted that the selectivity of these shunts is never completely achieved or is lost during follow-up,[16] and probably for these reasons, no major differences in clinical outcomes among these 2 types of shunt are found at medium- or long-term follow-up.[12] Nonshunt operations generally include esophageal transection or devascularization of the gastroesophageal junction.[17]

Although the data on the efficacy of these treatments are difficult to combine because of the heterogeneity of the patients studied, the different types of operations used, and the varying therapies used for supportive management, portal decompressive surgery and esophageal transection are highly effective in achieving hemostasis.[12,18] However, despite the success in controlling bleeding, the mortality of these patients is still high (approximately 45%–75%).[12,18] In addition, in patients surviving the bleeding episode, shunt surgery significantly increases the incidence of chronic or recurrent portal systemic encephalopathy (PSE),[12] and portacaval shunts alter vascular anatomy, which complicates future liver transplant surgery. The calibrated small-diameter portacaval H-graft shunt has reduced PSE in comparison with total PCS in the only randomized controlled trial (RCT) reported.[19]

TIPS

Few studies have compared TIPS with surgical techniques as a rescue therapy for variceal bleeding; 1 study by Rosemurgy and colleagues[20,21] compared TIPS with a surgical H-graft shunt in a total of 132 patients. The frequency of rebleeding was 16% in the TIPS group versus 3% in the surgery group. Thirty-day and total mortality were 15% versus 20%, and 43% versus 30% in the TIPS and surgery groups, respectively. The investigators of this study recommended surgery as the best treatment option. However, this study was not randomized and the stents used were not covered, a type of stent that has been shown to be associated with a lower incidence of TIPS dysfunction and a higher clinical efficacy than the bare stents.[22] In another study, Henderson and colleagues[23] randomized 140 patients with refractory variceal bleeding to distal splenorenal shunt or TIPS using bare stents. They did not find significant differences in rebleeding, incidence of hepatic encephalopathy, or in survival. In a single nonrandomized study, TIPS was shown to be superior to esophageal transaction in rebleeding (15% vs 26%) and 30-day mortality (42% vs 79%).[18] In these studies, most patients had enough liver reserve to be submitted to a surgical intervention, whereas patients with acute treatment failure usually had severe liver dysfunction. In addition, in the studies by Rosemurgy and colleagues[20,21] and Henderson and colleagues[23] the patients included had acute treatment failure or treatment failure in the prevention of rebleeding. Therefore the results observed in these studies probably do not reflect the real effect of rescue TIPS or rescue surgery in acute treatment failures.

The analysis of several uncontrolled series that have evaluated the use of TIPS exclusively in patients with acute treatment failure[24–27] confirmed that TIPS is highly successful in controlling bleeding (90%–100%). However, despite the control of bleeding, and as a consequence of multiple blood transfusions, repeated endoscopic treatments, and development of infections and of hepatic encephalopathy, a high proportion of these patients died of liver and multiorgan failure. It is therefore highly unlikely that the poor outcome of these patients may be changed by further improving the efficacy of rescue therapies. Therefore, strategies intended to improve the prognosis of these patients should focus on identifying those high-risk patients in whom standard therapy is likely to fail, and who are therefore candidates for more aggressive therapies early after the development of AVB.

TREATMENT STRATEGIES FOR HIGH-RISK PATIENTS

In patients with cirrhosis and AVB several factors,[1,28–35] such as Child-Pugh class and score, aspartate aminotransferase (AST) levels, shock at admission, presence of portal vein thrombosis, presence of hepatocellular carcinoma, active bleeding at endoscopy on admission, and hepatic venous pressure gradient (HVPG) of 20 mm Hg or more, have been shown to predict prognosis. One or a combination of these factors could help in classifying patients into different risk strata, making it possible to individualize the initial treatment of patients who experience an AVB episode. Possible modifications of the current recommended treatments of AVB that may be useful to improve the outcome of these high-risk patients are discussed later in this article.

Individualizing Drug Therapy

The usual dose of somatostatin in the treatment of AVB is a continuous infusion of 250 μg/h. Nonetheless, hemodynamic studies have shown that the reduction in portal pressure and azygos blood flow, a surrogate of blood flow through esophageal varices, is significantly higher with a dose of 500 μg/h.[36] An RCT[37] evaluated the efficacy of these 2 different doses. No significant differences were observed in relation to control of bleeding or in mortality. In this study, active bleeding at endoscopy was the only predictor of failure to control bleeding. A post hoc analysis of this high-risk subpopulation showed that patients receiving 500 μg/h of somatostatin had a significantly higher control of bleeding, a lower number of red blood transfusions, and better survival than those receiving 250 μg/h, suggesting that in high-risk patients (but not in the general population of patients with variceal bleeding), the 500 μg/h dose should be used. Another study[38] showed that terlipressin and the dose of 500 μg/h of somatostatin achieve a reduction in HVPG of 10% or more in a significantly higher proportion of patients than the dose of 250 μg/h of somatostatin. In this study, reduction in HVPG was even more pronounced with terlipressin than with 500 μg/h somatostatin (15% vs 10%), and a decrease in HVPG of more than 20% was observed in 36% of patients with terlipressin versus 5% with 500 μg/h somatostatin. Whether the higher reduction in HVPG obtained by 500 μg/h somatostatin, or even more by terlipressin, translates into a higher efficacy in controlling AVB must be evaluated in specifically designed studies in patients with a high risk of treatment failure. Confirmatory studies including exclusively high-risk patients are especially pertinent. Although the post hoc analysis of an RCT suggested that the addition of recombinant activated factor VII (rFVIIa), aimed at normalizing the coagulative defect of cirrhotic patients, improved the results of the standard treatment with drugs plus EBL in patients with moderate and advanced liver failure (stages B and C of the Child-Pugh classification),[39] these findings were not confirmed in a more recent trial specifically designed to test this issue in a high-risk population (defined in this study as patients with active bleeding at endoscopy and a Child-Pugh score ≥8 points).[40]

TIPS

TIPS is more effective than drugs or EBL in the control or prevention of variceal bleeding, but at an increase in cost and in the incidence of hepatic encephalopathy without improving survival.[41,42] As a consequence, in current practice TIPS is considered the rescue derivative therapy of choice in patients in whom medical and endoscopic treatment has failed.[3,4] However, as previously mentioned, treatment failure in the context of AVB is usually a desperate condition in which, despite the high success of TIPS, mortality due to liver failure is still high.

The paradigm of the use of TIPS only as a rescue treatment has recently been challenged by a study suggesting that, in high-risk patients, TIPS may be the initial treatment of preference.[33] In this RCT by Monescillo and colleagues,[33] early treatment with TIPS in high-risk patients, identified by an HVPG of 20 mm Hg or more,[32] improved prognosis in comparison with medical treatment. However, in this study, treatment administered in the medical arm was not the current standard of care,[33] and therefore it may be argued that the outcome of these patients was inferior to that expected now. In contrast, bare stents were used in the study by Monescillo and colleagues.[33] Polytetrafluoroethylene (PTFE)-covered stents are associated with a lower incidence of TIPS dysfunction and recurrence of portal hypertension–related complications.[22] Therefore, it is feasible that the study by Monescillo and colleagues[33] was unable to show the true potential of the early use of TIPS in improving the outcomes of high-risk variceal bleeders.

The clinical effect of the early use of TIPS in high-risk patients has been confirmed in a recent study[43] not yet published in full. In this study, 63 cirrhotic patients with AVB, defined as high risk according to simple and readily available clinical variables, were randomized (within 24 hours of admission) to receive TIPS using PTFE-covered stents (within the first 72 hours after admission), or to continue receiving vasoactive drugs plus EBL, followed after 3 to 5 days by nadolol or propranolol plus mononitrate plus EBL. Patients treated with early PTFE TIPS had a significant reduction in failure to control bleeding, and of variceal rebleeding, than those treated with drugs plus EBL. In addition, and more importantly, the use of early TIPS was associated with a significant and marked reduction in mortality. Six-week mortality was reduced from 33% in the drug plus EBL group to 4% in the early TIPS group. The major effect in mortality was in the population at a higher risk of death (ie, Child-Pugh C patients). The beneficial effect on survival was observed despite offering rescue PTFE TIPS to those patients in the drug plus EBL group with treatment failure.

The concept that the use of an early derivative procedure may be a good therapeutic alternative in the treatment of AVB has been proposed by Orloff and colleagues.[44] This study showed superior control of bleeding and better survival with the performance of an emergent portacaval shunt within 8 hours of admission as the initial treatment of bleeding in comparison with the use of a medical approach (intravenous vasopressin and balloon tamponade).[44] However, this study has been criticized because of the

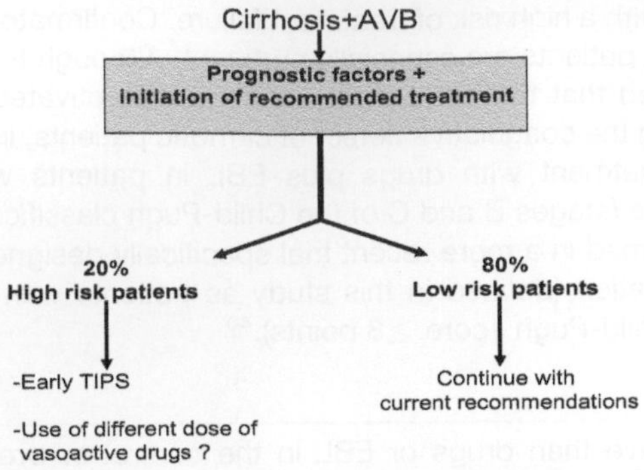

Fig. 2. The possible treatment strategy of AVB according to different risk strata.

great difficulty in applying this approach in clinical practice. Nevertheless, the results of this trial are in accordance with more recent findings of the early use of TIPS.

SUMMARY

Current recommendations for the treatment of AVB are applied homogenously to all cirrhotic patients without considering special characteristic that may influence the outcome of these treatments.[3,4] However, despite the application of these gold-standard treatments, 10% to 15% of cirrhotic patients still have treatment failure.[1,4] Despite the high success of rescue TIPS in controlling bleeding in treatment failures, the mortality of patients in whom the initial approach failed is high due to liver failure. It is possible that in the near future, patients may be treated "à la carte" (**Fig. 2**). Indeed, in high-risk patients, more aggressive therapies with early PTFE TIPS may be the treatment of choice.[42,43] To achieve this goal it is important to refine our capacity to identify populations of patients with different risks.

ACKNOWLEDGMENTS

The authors are grateful for the review of this manuscript by Gautam Mehta, MRCP.

REFERENCES

1. D'Amico G, de Franchis R. Upper digestive bleeding in cirrhosis. Post-therapeutic outcome and prognostic indicators. Hepatology 2003;38:599–612.
2. D'Amico G, Pagliaro L, Bosch J. Pharmacological treatment of portal hypertension: an evidence-based approach. Semin Liver Dis 1999;19:475–505.
3. de Franchis R. Evolving consensus in portal hypertension report of the Baveno IV Consensus Workshop on methodology of diagnosis and therapy in portal hypertension. J Hepatol 2005;43:167–76.
4. Garcia-Tsao G, Sanyal AJ, Grace ND, et al. Prevention and management of gastroesophageal varices and variceal hemorrhage in cirrhosis. Hepatology 2007;46:922–38.
5. Banares R, Albillos A, Rincon D, et al. Endoscopic treatment versus endoscopic plus pharmacologic treatment for acute variceal bleeding: a meta-analysis. Hepatology 2002;35:609–15.
6. D'Amico G, Criscuoli V, Filì D, et al. Meta-analysis of trials for variceal bleeding. Hepatology 2002;36(4):1023–4.

7. Chojkier M, Conn HO. Esophageal tamponade in the treatment of bleeding varices. A decadel progress report. Dig Dis Sci 1980;25:267–72.
8. Hunt PS, Korman MG, Hansky J, et al. An 8-year prospective experience with balloon tamponade in emergency control of bleeding esophageal varices. Dig Dis Sci 1982;27:413–6.
9. Fort E, Sautereau D, Silvain C, et al. A randomized trial of terlipressin plus nitroglycerin vs. balloon tamponade in the control of acute variceal hemorrhage. Hepatology 1990;11:678–81.
10. Paquet KJ, Feussner H. Endoscopic sclerosis and esophageal balloon tamponade in acute hemorrhage from esophagogastric varices: a prospective controlled randomized trial. Hepatology 1985;5:580–3.
11. Pitcher JL. Safety and effectiveness of the modified Sengstaken-Blakemore tube: a prospective study. Gastroenterology 1971;61:291–8.
12. D'Amico G, Pagliaro L, Bosch J. The treatment of portal hypertension: a meta-analytic review. Hepatology 1995;22:332–54.
13. Hubmann R, Bodlaj G, Czompo M, et al. The use of self-expanding metal stents to treat acute esophageal variceal bleeding. Endoscopy 2006;38: 896–901.
14. Benko L, Danis J, Czompo M, et al. DSC examination of the oesophagus after two different self-expandable stents implantation. J Therm Anal Calorim 2006;83: 715–20.
15. Hogan B, Path D, Burrougs A, et al. Use of the SX-Ella self-expanding mesh metal stent in the management of complex variceal hemorrhage: initial experience in a single centre. J. of Hepatology 2009;50:S86–7.
16. Belghiti J, Grenier P, Nouel O, et al. Long-term loss of Warren's shunt selectivity. Angiographic demonstration. Arch Surg 1981;116(9):1121–4.
17. Terblanche J. The surgeon's role in the management of portal hypertension. Ann Surg 1989;209(4):381–95.
18. Jalan R, John TG, Redhead DN, et al. A comparative study of emergency transjugular intrahepatic portosystemic stent-shunt and esophageal transection in the management of uncontrolled variceal hemorrhage. Am J Gastroenterol 1995;90: 1932–7.
19. Sarfeh IJ, Rypins EB. Partial versus total portocaval shunt in alcoholic cirrhosis. Results of a prospective, randomized clinical trial. Ann Surg 1994;219:353–61.
20. Rosemurgy AS, Goode SE, Zwiebel BR, et al. A prospective trial of transjugular intrahepatic portasystemic stent shunts versus small-diameter prosthetic H-graft portacaval shunts in the treatment of bleeding varices. Ann Surg 1996;224: 378–84.
21. Rosemurgy AS, Serafini FM, Zweibel BR, et al. Transjugular intrahepatic portosystemic shunt vs. small-diameter prosthetic H-graft portacaval shunt: extended follow-up of an expanded randomized prospective trial. J Gastrointest Surg 2000;4:589–97.
22. Bureau C, Garcia-Pagan JC, Pomier-layrargues G, et al. Improved clinical outcome using polytetrafluoroethylene-coated stents for TIPS: results of a randomized study. Gastroenterology 2004;126(2):469–75.
23. Henderson JM, Boyer TD, Kutne MH, et al. Distal splenorenal shunt versus transjugular intrahepatic portal systematic shunt for variceal bleeding: a randomized trial. Gastroenterology 2006;130(6):1643–51.
24. Gerbes AL, Gulberg V, Waggershauser T, et al. Transjugular intrahepatic portosystemic shunt (TIPS) for variceal bleeding in portal hypertension: comparison of emergency and elective interventions. Dig Dis Sci 1998;43:2463–9.

25. Chau TN, Patch D, Chan YW, et al. "Salvage" transjugular intrahepatic portosystemic shunts: gastric fundal compared with esophageal variceal bleeding. Gastroenterology 1998;114:981.
26. LaBerge JM, Somberg KA, Lake JR, et al. Two-year outcome following transjugular intrahepatic portosystemic shunt for variceal bleeding: results in 90 patients. Gastroenterology 1995;108:1143.
27. Sanyal AJ, Freedman AM, Luketic VA, et al. Transjugular intrahepatic portosystemic shunts for patients with active variceal hemorrhage unresponsive to sclerotherapy. Gastroenterology 1996;111:138.
28. Lecleire S, Di Fiore F, Merle V, et al. Acute upper gastrointestinal bleeding in patients with liver cirrhosis and in noncirrhotic patients: epidemiology and predictive factors of mortality in a prospective multicenter population-based study. J Clin Gastroenterol 2005;39:321–7.
29. Thomopoulos K, Theocharis G, Mimidis K, et al. Improved survival of patients presenting with acute variceal bleeding. Prognostic indicators of short- and long-term mortality. Dig Liver Dis 2006;38:899–904.
30. Bambha Kiran, Ray Kim W, Pedersen Rachel A, et al. Predictors of rebleeding and mortality following acute variceal hemorrhage in patients with cirrhosis. Gut 2008;57:814–20.
31. Ripoll C, Bañares R, Rincón D, et al. Influence of hepatic venous pressure gradient on the prediction of survival of patients with cirrhosis in the MELD Era. Hepatology 2005;42(4):793–801.
32. Moitinho E, Escorsell A, Bandi JC, et al. Prognostic value of early measurements of portal pressure in acute variceal bleeding. Gastroenterology 1999;117:626–31.
33. Monescillo A, Martinez-Lagares F, Ruiz-del-Arbol L, et al. Influence of portal hypertension and its early decompression by TIPS placement on the outcome of variceal bleeding. Hepatology 2004;40:793–801.
34. Avgerinos A, Armonis A, Stefanidis G, et al. Sustained rise of portal pressure after sclerotherapy, but not band ligation, in acute variceal bleeding in cirrhosis. Hepatology 2004;39:1623–30.
35. Abraldes JG, Villanueva C, Bañares R, et al. Hepatic venous pressure gradient and prognosis in patients with acute variceal bleeding treated with pharmacologic and endoscopic therapy. J Hepatol 2008;48:229–36.
36. Cirera I, Feu F, Luca A, et al. Effects of bolus injections and continuous infusions of somatostatin and placebo in patients with cirrhosis: a double-blind hemodynamic investigation. Hepatology 1995;22(1):106–11.
37. Moitinho E, Planas R, Bañares R, et al. Multicenter randomized controlled trial comparing different schedules of somatostatin in the treatment of acute variceal bleeding. J Hepatol 2001;35:712–8.
38. Villanueva C, Piqueras M, Aracil C, et al. A randomized controlled trial comparing ligation and sclerotherapy as emergency endoscopic treatment added to somatostatin in acute variceal bleeding. J Hepatol 2006;45:560–7.
39. Bosch J, Thabut D, Bendtsen F, et al. Recombinant factor VIIa for upper gastrointestinal bleeding in patients with cirrhosis: a randomized, double-blind trial. Gastroenterology 2004;127:1123–30.
40. Bosch J, Thabut D, Albillos A, et al. Recombinant factor VIIA (RFVIIA) for active variceal bleeding in patients with advanced cirrhosis: a randomized controlled trial. Hepatology 2008;47(5):1604–14.
41. Escorsell A, Bañares R, García-Pagán JC, et al. TIPS versus drug therapy in preventing variceal rebleeding in advanced cirrhosis: a randomized controlled trial. Hepatology 2002;35(2):385–92.

42. Khan S, Tudur Smith C, Williamson P, et al. Portosystemic shunts versus endoscopic therapy for variceal rebleeding in patients with cirrhosis. Cochrane Database Syst Rev 2006;4:CD000553.
43. Garcia-Pagan JC, Caca K, Bureau C, et-al. An early decision for PTFE-TIPS improves survival in high risk cirrhotic patient admitted with an acute variceal bleeding. A multicenter RCT. Hepatology 2008;48(4):373A.
44. Orloff MJ, Bell RH Jr, Orloff MS, et al. Prospective randomized trial of emergency portacaval shunt and emergency medical therapy in unselected cirrhotic patients with bleeding varices. Hepatology 1994;20(4 Pt 1):863–72.

The Role of Endoscopy in Secondary Prophylaxis of Esophageal Varices

Gin-Ho Lo, MD[a,b,*]

KEYWORDS

- Variceal rebleeding • Endoscopy • Sclerotherapy
- Banding ligation • Endoscopic therapy

Esophageal variceal hemorrhage is a devastating complication of portal hypertension, associated with a high morbidity and mortality.[1] Once acute bleeding is successfully controlled, rebleeding may occur in approximately two-thirds of patients if further preventive measures are not taken. Several factors have been noted to be associated with the occurrence of variceal rebleeding; including portal pressure, poor liver reserve, sizes of varices, treatment modalities of acute bleeding, infection, and portal vein thrombosis (**Box 1**).[2–10] Except for moribund patients, measures should be taken to reduce variceal rebleeding episodes to improve patients' survival. The time frame of variceal rebleeding can be divided into very early rebleeding (within 5 days of acute bleeding), early rebleeding (within 6 weeks of acute bleeding), and delayed rebleeding.[11] By definition, prevention of variceal rebleeding starts on day 6. The armamentarium for the prevention of variceal rebleeding includes surgical shunt therapy, endoscopic therapy, pharmacotherapy, and transjugular intrahepatic portosystemic stent shunt (TIPS). Although shunt operation and TIPS are highly effective in the reduction of variceal rebleeding, they may be associated with hepatic encephalopathy or other serious morbidities. These 2 methods are reserved for endoscopic and medical therapy failure. Endoscopic therapy has evolved from sclerotherapy to banding ligation over the past 15 years, and emerges as an important weapon in the fight against variceal rebleeding. This review focuses on the role of endoscopy in secondary prophylaxis of esophageal varices. The available endoscopic modalities to prevent variceal rebleeding are shown in **Box 2**.

[a] Department of Medical Education, Digestive Center, E-DA Hospital, 1, Yi-Da Road, Kaohsiung County 824, Taiwan, Republic of China
[b] I-Shou University, Kaohsiung, Taiwan, Republic of China
* Department of Medical Education, Digestive Center, E-DA Hospital, 1, Yi-Da Road, Kaohsiung County 824, Taiwan, Republic of China.
E-mail address: ghlo@kimo.com

Clin Liver Dis 14 (2010) 307–323
doi:10.1016/j.cld.2010.03.009
liver.theclinics.com
1089-3261/10/$ – see front matter

Box 1
Factors possibly affecting variceal rebleeding rates in patients receiving endoscopic therapy

Child-Pugh class

Active bleeding at endoscopy

Bacterial infection

Variceal size

Portal pressure, variceal pressure

Presence of paraesophageal varices

Presence of hepatocellular carcinoma

Presence of portal thrombosis

Continued alcohol use

Methods of endoscopic therapy

Endoscopist's skill

Treatment intervals

ENDOSCOPIC INJECTION SCLEROTHERAPY

Endoscopic injection sclerotherapy (EIS) using quinine as a sclerosant was first introduced by Crafoord and Frenckner, two Swedish surgeons, in 1939.[12] Subsequently other sclerosants such as sodium morrhuate, podidocanol, ethanolamine, alcohol, and sodium tetradecyl sulfate were more widely used. The mechanisms of EIS are via injection of sclerosants resulting in tissue necrosis and finally causing fibrosis, leading to obliteration of varices. The techniques of EIS vary widely among different clinicians. Some doctors use free-hand injections, others prefer to incorporate a balloon onto the distal end of the endoscope to compress the varices following injections.[13] The optimal dose of sclerosants is also unknown, ranging of from 1 mL to 50 mL having been employed. In general, use of alcohol at 50% concentration may cause painful sensation and severe ulcerations, thus only a small amount of alcohol can be injected during each session. Although some studies tried to compare the effectiveness between varying sclerosants,[14] it is difficult to draw a final conclusion. The treatment can be injected either intravariceally or paravariceally. Paravariceal injection using a large volume of polidocanol to form a protective fibrosis layer around varices

Box 2
Endoscopic methods for preventing variceal rebleeding

Endoscopic injection sclerotherapy (EIS)

Endoscopic variceal ligation (EVL)

Synchronous combination of EIS and EVL

Metachronous combination of EIS and EVL

Metachronous combination of EVL and argon plasma coagulation

Endoscopic clipping

Tissue adhesive

was generally adopted by European gastroenterologists. The treatment interval varied between a few days to weeks.[15] A shorter interval might shorten the duration required to achieve variceal obliteration, resulting in a reduced frequency of early rebleeding, whereas the incidence of postsclerotherapy ulcers might increase. EIS appeared to be uniformly beneficial, regardless of the variation in techniques.[16] In the full-blown era of surgery, EIS was not regarded as a useful tool to prevent variceal rebleeding and lapsed into obscurity. In 1973, Johnston and Rodgers[17] reported that EIS could achieve a satisfactory effect in preventing variceal rebleeding, leading to reduced mortality. These results ignited enthusiasm for EIS akin to a renaissance of EIS. Since then, EIS has been widely employed to prevent variceal rebleeding up until the advent of endoscopic variceal ligation (EVL).

Four widely cited studies of EIS for the treatment of esophageal varices, the South African trial, the Los Angeles trial, the Copenhagen trial, and the King's College trial, were published between1983 and 1985.[18–21] Reduced variceal rebleeding with EIS was shown in 2 studies and improved survival was shown in only 1 study. Recurrent variceal bleeding reduced from 54% to 82% of the control groups to 48% to 55% after repeated sessions of EIS.[22] However, several local and systemic complications may arise after EIS.[13,23–26] These complications can be classified as local: esophageal ulcers, ulcer bleeding, and esophageal stricture; cardiovascular and respiratory: pleural effusion, adult respiratory distress syndrome, and pericarditis; and systemic: fever, bacteremia, spontaneous bacterial peritonitis, distant embolism, and distant abscess. It is impossible to predict what kind of complications may be encountered in which patients receiving EIS. Among them, bacteremia, postsclerotherapy esophageal ulcer bleeding, and stricture are the most frequent adverse events.[23–26] The main cause of these hazardous complications is usually an extensive wall necrosis induced by an incorrect injection technique, too much sclerosant being injected, or a high concentration of the sclerosant.[27] Mortality directly resulting from post-EIS complications may be noted in 2% of patients. Meta-analyses of the trials published between 1982 and 1991, comparing EIS with "nonactive" treatment, showed that patients treated with long-term EIS had a significantly lower rebleeding rate (pooled odds ratio 0.57; 95% confidence interval 0.45–0.71) and better survival than those who received only nonactive treatment (pooled odds ratio 0.72; 95% confidence interval 0.57–0.90).[28,29] Among patients receiving endoscopic therapy, the variceal rebleeding rate could only be significantly reduced after variceal obliteration. However, in general more than 5 sessions are required to achieve variceal obliteration in a patient presenting with severe esophageal varices. In one study, a mean of 10 sessions of EIS was required to achieve variceal obliteration[30]; this constitutes another drawback of EIS.

After initial obliteration of varices, regular surveillance at intervals of 6 months to detect recurrent varices is required. On the other hand, Kitano and colleagues[31] adopted a different approach to prevent variceal recurrence by injecting 1 to 2 mL of sclerosant into the residual mucosa at the later stage of repeated EIS to produce superficial ulcers in the lower esophagus. These ulcers healed with reepithelization and submucosal fibrosis, leaving no area for the development of new varices. Among 141 patients receiving this EIS method, no variceal recurrence was noted after a median follow-up of 16 months. Among 438 patients treated with EIS, Kitano and Baatar[32] observed that only 10.5% had recurrent bleeding during the median follow-up of 700 days. The main side effect was a high incidence of mild esophageal stricture. Severe stricture requiring bougie dilatation was rarely encountered. Despite its success, this unique EIS technique was abandoned by endoscopists because of its complexity.

COMPARISON OF EIS AND MEDICAL THERAPY

Both β-blockers and EIS were important and popular modalities in the prevention of variceal rebleeding during the 1980s. Studies comparing EIS and β-blockers were widely performed. A meta-analysis of 9 trials comparing β-blockers with EIS showed a significant reduction of rebleeding in favor of EIS (pooled odds ratio 0.64, 95% confidence interval 0.48–0.85).[33] However, significantly more complications were encountered in patients receiving EIS, while survival was similar between both therapies. Furthermore, a controlled trial showed that the combination of nadolol and isosorbide mononitrate (ISMN) was superior to EIS in the reduction of variceal rebleeding.[34] It was thus recommended that β-blockers rather than EIS should be the first choice to prevent recurrent variceal bleeding in the 1990s.[35]

ENDOSCOPIC VARICEAL LIGATION

In 1989, Stiegmann and Goff[36] introduced the application of EVL to treat esophageal varices. In contrast to the use of chemical action evoked by EIS, EVL obliterates varices by causing mechanical strangulation with rubber bands, just like its use in the treatment of hemorrhoids. Owing to its action on the suctioned, entrapped varices, the main reaction is usually limited over the superficial esophageal mucosa. In general, one varix is ligated with 1 or 2 rubber bands during each session. Different from a variety of technical variations practiced in EIS, the techniques of EVL appear unanimously similar except for the treatment interval. Initially, a single ligator associated with an overtube was employed to ligate varices. Subsequently, the multiband ligator was invented to avoid the use of an overtube and its associated complications. No significant differences in efficacy exist between these ligators. The use of endoloop is similar to application of EVL.[37] After the application of rubber bands over esophageal varices, the ligated tissues with rubber bands may fall off within a few days (range: 1–10 days). Following the sloughing of varices, shallow esophageal ulcers are ubiquitous at ligated sites and esophageal varices become smaller in diameter. The ligation-induced ulcers are shallower, have greater surface area, and heal more rapidly than those caused by EIS.[38] The complications of EVL include esophageal laceration or perforation (mostly due to trauma of the overtube), transient dysphagia, retrosternal pain, esophageal stricture, transient accentuation of portal hypertensive gastropathy, ulcer bleeding, and bacteremia.[39]

COMPARISON OF EIS AND EVL

Between 1992 and 1994, 7 studies including 4 randomized trials comparing EIS and EVL in the prevention of variceal rebleeding appeared in the literature.[40–43] Most of these studies proved that EVL was superior to EIS in terms of reducing rebleeding rates and complication rates, but only 2 trials showed better survival with EVL.[40,43] In 1995 Laine and Cook[44] performed a meta-analysis of these reports and showed that rebleeding from esophageal varices, mortality, esophageal strictures, and treatment sessions required for variceal obliteration were significantly reduced in patients receiving EVL compared with those receiving EIS. The second meta-analysis including 13 articles was performed in 1999 by de Franchis and Primignani[28], and revealed a strong benefit for EVL in decreasing variceal rebleeding (pooled odds ratio 0.46, 95% confidence interval 0.35–0.60) and similar survival between patients treated with EIS and those treated with EVL. The mean sessions required to achieve variceal obliteration was reduced from 5.4 in patients receiving EIS to 3.6 in patients receiving EVL. Recurrent variceal bleeding was reduced from between 8% and 53% in the EIS groups to between 2% and 36% of patients receiving EVL. The high incidence of esophageal stricture and ulcer bleeding associated with EIS was significantly reduced with EVL. A comparative study by the author's group demonstrated that bacteremia and infectious sequelae after EIS were 5 to 10 times greater than after EVL.[45] Therefore, for all the aforementioned reasons, EVL is the recommended endoscopic treatment for the management of bleeding esophageal varices.[46] The main disadvantage of EVL is possibly a higher frequency of recurrent varices.[47–49] Fortunately, those recurrent varices can usually be treated with repeated ligation. Moreover, the recurrence after EVL did not lead to a higher risk of rebleeding or require more endoscopic treatments.[49] A large meta-analysis did not prove that EVL-treated patients were predisposed to develop recurrent varices.[28] Similar to EIS, the appropriate interval between sessions of EVL has not yet been determined. Most endoscopists and scholars advocate an interval of 1 or 2 weeks,[40–42,50] whereas the author believes that an interval of 3 to 4 weeks is more suitable, given that unhealed ulcers induced by ligation are frequently noted within 2 weeks of ligation. EVL at a longer interval does not result in a higher rebleeding rate. In fact, in the author's experience the rebleeding rate was generally lower than those of other reports.[43] A study from Japan demonstrated that EVL performed once every 2 months was better than EVL performed once every 2 weeks regarding overall rates of variceal recurrence.[51] Because the rebleeding rate of patients receiving endoscopic therapy could only be significantly reduced in those who achieve variceal obliteration within a short period, EVL performed at intervals of 2 months in the prevention of variceal rebleeding may be inappropriate. The other retrospective study from the United States also revealed that an interbanding interval of 3 weeks or longer was associated with a lower rebleeding rate.[52] The optimal interval of EVL in the prevention of variceal rebleeding awaits further evaluation. On the other hand, Ramirez and colleagues[53] conducted a study showing that as many rubber bands as possible placed per session could not achieve variceal obliteration with fewer sessions, compared with patients receiving up to a maximum of 6 bands in one session.

Apart from differences in effectiveness and safety in the reduction of rebleeding, esophageal motility was also demonstrated to be significantly influenced by EIS but not by EVL.[54,55] It therefore appears that EIS should be abandoned following the introduction of EVL in the prevention of variceal rebleeding, except for endoscopists who are specialized in EIS with comparably low rebleeding rates and complications to EVL. The comparison between EIS and EVL is shown in **Table 1**. Due to the superiority of EVL over EIS, the role of EIS in the prevention of variceal rebleeding has been nearly completely replaced by EVL.[27,56]

COMPARISON OF EVL AND MEDICAL THERAPY

The combination of β-blockers and ISMN proving superiority over EIS in reducing variceal rebleeding evokes interest in evaluating whether this combination is comparable with EVL.[34] Up to now, there have been 5 controlled trials comparing the combination of nadolol and ISMN with EVL in the prevention of variceal rebleeding (**Table 2**).[57–61] These trials had 3 different results; 2 studies showed that EVL was superior, another showed that pharmacologic therapy was superior, and the other 2 showed equivalent efficacy for both therapies. It is difficult to draw a conclusion about which therapy is superior. As mentioned earlier, one of the determining factors of variceal rebleeding is severity of cirrhosis. The operators' expertise in EVL, etiology of cirrhosis, and dosage of portal hypotensive drugs also may have an impact on the rebleeding rates. Meta-analysis of the first 4 studies showed similar survival between pharmacologic

Table 1
Comparison between EIS and EVL

	EIS	EVL
Mechanisms	Chemical	Mechanical
Treatment sessions required to variceal obliteration	More sessions	Fewer
Rates of variceal obliteration	Similar	Similar
Complications	More common	Fewer
Posttreatment ulcers	Less common but deeper	More common but shallower
Posttreatment ulcer bleeding	More common	Less common
Esophageal stricture	More common	Less common
Infectious sequelae	More common	Less common
Impaired esophageal motility	Frequently	Rarely
Rebleeding rates	More common	Fewer
Variceal recurrence	Less common	More common
Prevalence of paraesophageal varices	Less common	More common
Survival	Similar or worse	Similar or better

therapy and EVL,[62] suggesting that either medication with nadolol plus ISMN or EVL can be used to prevent esophageal variceal rebleeding. Previous reports generally observed only a short duration. The author's group extended their study to compare the long-term effectiveness and survival of EVL with nadolol and ISMN in the prevention of rebleeding from esophageal varices. The study demonstrated that EVL was definitely better than combination drug therapy in terms of prevention of rebleeding from esophageal varices. Blood requirements were slightly lower in the patients who underwent repeated EVL than in those who received nadolol plus ISMN. On the other hand, the survival in patients treated with combination drug therapy appeared to be better than in those treated with repeated EVL.[63] Nonetheless, β-blockers had to be discontinued in up to 25% of patients because of adverse effects. EVL is the preferred approach among those patients in whom β-blockers fail or are intolerable.

ENDOSCOPIC CLIPPING

The endoscopic clipping apparatus was originally developed by Hayashi and colleagues[64] in 1975, and was further improved by Hachisu[65] in 1988. Endoscopic

Table 2
Controlled studies of EVL versus nadolol + ISMN to prevent variceal rebleeding

Authors	No. of Patients	Therapy	Rebleeding (%)	Complication (%)	Mortality (%)
Villanueva et al[57]	72/72	EVL/N+I	44/28[a]	12/3[a]	42/32
Lo et al[58]	61/60	EVL/N+I	20/42[a]	17/19	25/13
Patch et al[59]	51/51	EVL/P+I	54/44	14/20	22/32
Romero et al[60]	57/52	EVL+EIS/N+I	40/37	49/46	19/20
Sarin et al[61]	71/66	EVL/P+I	22/37[a]	33/25	8/6

Abbreviations: N+I, nadolol + ISMN; ISMN, isosorbide mononitrate; P, propranolol; EVL, endoscopic variceal ligation.
[a] Significant difference.

clipping is widely used in the management of bleeding ulcers. This device has the advantage of targeting vessels with minimal damage to the surrounding tissue. Its application in the management of bleeding varices has been rarely addressed. Yol and colleagues[66] performed a controlled trial to compare endoscopic clipping and EVL in the management of bleeding esophageal varices and eventual variceal obliteration. The results showed that the mean number of sessions required to achieve variceal obliteration was significantly lower in patients treated with endoscopic clipping than in those receiving EVL (3 vs 4). Moreover, esophageal ulcers were noted in 90% of patients treated with EVL, whereas no ulcers were found in the endoscopic clipping group. The rebleeding rates were slightly lower in patients receiving endoscopic clipping (15%) than the figure of 33% achieved by EVL. Although endoscopic clipping appeared to have fewer complications and was more effective than EVL in achieving variceal obliteration, the study was flawed with a very small sample size. During clip application, caution must be taken to avoid gouging a varix with the pointed corners of an open clip that may elicit bleeding. The application of endoscopic clipping to prevent variceal rebleeding awaits further investigation.

TISSUE ADHESIVE (HISTOACRYL INJECTION)

Histoacryl injection is widely employed in the management of gastric variceal bleeding and acute bleeding from esophageal varices.[67,68] The use of histoacryl injection in the prevention of variceal rebleeding from esophageal varices is rarely addressed.[69,70] Some studies suggested that combined histoacryl injection and EIS is superior to EIS alone in the reduction of early variceal rebleeding.[68] However, there have been no trials comparing histoacryl injection with EVL, which is now accepted as the endoscopic treatment of choice for esophageal variceal rebleeding. A study comparing histoacryl injection with propranolol in the prevention of gastroesophageal variceal rebleeding disclosed that both therapies were equivalent in the prevention of variceal rebleeding but that histoacryl injection was associated with more complications.[71] Based on these studies, histoacryl injection cannot be advocated as a tool to prevent esophageal variceal rebleeding.

SYNCHRONOUS COMBINATION OF EIS AND EVL

Combination of endoscopic therapies to manage esophageal varices has been a focus of interest for endoscopists. In the context of different action mechanisms of EIS and EVL, combining EIS and EVL theoretically achieves eradication of varices more rapidly. It has been noted that paraesophageal varices could be obliterated by EIS but not by EVL.[72] The combination of EIS and EVL is potentially able to reduce variceal recurrence after obliteration. The combination of EIS and EVL can be synchronous or metachronous. Synchronous combination means that sclerosants are injected into ligated varices during the same treatment session, whereas metachronous usually means that EIS is performed on small residual varices after repeated EVL of large varices. Between 1996 and 2000, 7 studies were performed to investigate the potential benefits of mostly synchronous combination with EIS, and a meta-analysis of these studies was performed by Singh and colleagues[73] in 2002. Combination therapy achieved significantly higher variceal obliteration than EVL alone; however, the overall rebleeding rate with EVL alone was 22%, which did not differ significantly from that of combination therapy, 20%. The survival was also similar between both methods of treatment. Moreover, combination therapy lengthened the treatment time and was associated with a higher complication rate of esophageal stricture. Hou and colleagues[74] tried to ligate varices initially, then used sclerotherapy and finally ligation once again during a treatment session, a so-called sandwich method. The results showed that combination could further reduce variceal rebleeding as compared with treatment with EVL alone. However, this method is somewhat complicated and is thus not imitated by other endoscopists. In Japan, some endoscopists adopted EIS followed by immediate EVL, which required fewer treatment sessions and fewer sclerosants to achieve variceal obliteration than patients treated with EIS alone.[75] However, there were no differences in variceal recurrence, variceal rebleeding, and complication rates between the 2 procedures. Because EIS has been replaced by EVL in the prevention of variceal rebleeding, these trials cannot be regarded as appropriate nowadays. Thus, the synchronous combination of EVL and EIS has been discarded.

METACHRONOUS COMBINATION OF EIS AND EVL

After repeated EVL, small residual varices cannot be further ligated, but they may recur. Thus, EIS with low-dose sclerosants following repeated EVL was developed to reduce variceal recurrence. Several trials have shown that metachronous combination therapy with EIS and EVL could reduce the variceal recurrence or even reduce incidence of variceal rebleeding as compared with that treated with EVL or EIS alone.[76–78] Thus, metachronous combination therapy with EIS and EVL is more favored than the synchronous combination. However, 1 or 2 further sessions of EIS treatment are required to enhance the efficacy.

On the other hand, Hashizume and colleagues[79] treated patients with first one session of EVL followed by repeated sessions of EIS. The 3-year cumulative variceal recurrence was remarkably high, 91% in those receiving combination therapy compared with 35% in those receiving EIS alone. Thus, this kind of metachronous combination therapy is not advocated.

To reduce variceal recurrence, Monici and colleagues[80] tried to apply microwave coagulation in patients receiving repeated EVL. The results disclosed that addition of microwaves reduced variceal recurrence to 17%, while addition of EIS had a recurrent rate of 27%. Cipolletta and colleagues[81] adopted argon plasma coagulation (APC) following variceal obliteration achieved by EVL. Their study demonstrated that variceal recurrence could be reduced from 43% in patients receiving EVL alone to 0% in patients receiving argon plasma as a "consolidation therapy" of repeated EVL. Transient fever, dysphagia, and retrosternal discomfort were frequently encountered, though not severe. It seems that the addition of sclerotherapy, microwaves, or argon plasma following variceal obliteration achieved by EVL could effectively reduce variceal recurrence. However, the combination of EVL and microwaves or argon plasma requires controlled studies before it can be universally recommended.[82]

COMBINED EIS AND MEDICAL THERAPY

The combination of endoscopic therapy and drug therapy for portal hypertension is intriguing. Several reasons support the addition of drug therapy during endoscopic therapy. First, the rebleeding rate remains high after endoscopic therapy, especially before variceal obliteration is achieved.[1,2,8,10,83] The rebleeding rate is about 30% to 50% in patients treated with EIS and 20% to 40% in patients treated with EVL. Second, portal hypertensive gastropathy may develop or be accentuated after endoscopic therapy.[37,84–86]. An increased incidence of gastric variceal bleeding after endoscopic therapy has also been noted.[43,86] Third, portal pressure was noted to be elevated in approximately 70% of patients in whom variceal obliteration was achieved by either EIS or EVL.[87,88] Fourth, variceal recurrence is very common after variceal obliteration achieved by endoscopic therapy.[47–49] It is hopefully anticipated that all of these undesirable or untoward effects by endoscopic therapy could be abolished or alleviated by drug therapy.[10] Several studies were performed to compare the combination of propranolol plus EIS with propranolol or EIS alone.[89,90] Most studies did not show a benefit of combination with EIS and propranolol over single therapy. The variceal rebleeding rates and complications were similar between the 2 treatments in these studies. Meta-analysis of the 10 studies between 1986 and 1992 suggested that the combined treatment with EIS and propranolol was significantly better than EIS alone in preventing rebleeding (pooled odds ratio 0.65, 95% confidence interval 0.46–0.92), but with similar survival in both modalities.[91] After the introduction of EVL, the combination of EIS and drugs in the prevention of variceal rebleeding has been used only rarely.

COMBINED EVL AND MEDICAL THERAPY

In contrast to the enthusiasm shown for EIS plus β-blockers, the use of EVL and β-blockers in the prevention of variceal rebleeding has not been extensively studied. In view of the superiority of EVL over EIS and nadolol over propranolol, the author's group performed a trial combining EVL with nadolol and sucralfate compared with EVL alone for the prevention of variceal rebleeding.[92] The use of sucralfate was to reduce potential ulcer bleeding provoked by EVL. After a median follow-up of 21 months, the study showed that combination of nadolol, sucralfate, and EVL was superior to EVL alone in terms of variceal rebleeding rates (12% vs 29%) and variceal recurrence (26% vs 50%). It was presumed that the benefits of combination therapy were primarily from nadolol rather than sucralfate, because the incidence of ulcer bleeding during the course of EVL was appreciably low. A similar study by de la Pena and colleagues[93] also consistently showed that combination of EVL and β-blockers was superior to EVL alone in reducing variceal rebleeding as well as in prevention of variceal recurrence (**Table 3**). However, their patients treated with EVL plus nadolol had a higher frequency of complications, mostly caused by the use of β-blockers.

On the other hand, it is still unknown whether EVL could enhance the efficacy of β-blockers plus ISMN to prevent recurrent variceal bleeding. The author's group has performed such a study, whose results demonstrated that combined EVL with drug therapy had a variceal rebleeding rate of 28%, which was marginally significantly lower than the 48% achieved in patients treated with drug therapy only ($P = .05$).[94] A similar study from Spain with a short-term follow-up showed that the addition of EVL to pharmacologic therapy did not reduce the frequency of variceal rebleeding but had a higher frequency of severe complications requiring hospitalization.[95] A recent meta-analysis including 1860 patients from 23 studies performed between 1980 and 2007 found that combination endoscopic (either EIS or EVL) and drug therapy reduced overall rebleeding and variceal rebleeding more than endoscopic therapy alone or β-blocker therapy alone.[96] Combination therapy also reduced variceal recurrence but did not

Table 3
Controlled trials of EVL versus EVL + nadolol to prevent variceal rebleeding

Authors	No. of Patients	Therapy	Rebleeding (%)	Complication (%)	Mortality (%)
Lo et al[92]	62/60	EVL/EVL+N	29/12[a]	8/11	32/17
de la Pena et al[93]	37/43	EVL/EVL+N	38/14[a]	3/33[a]	11/11

Abbreviations: N, nadolol; EVL, endoscopic variceal ligation.
[a] Significant difference.

significantly reduce mortality. As a consequence, combination therapy for EVL and β-blockers is preferable to EVL alone in the prevention of variceal rebleeding.

Based on these studies, experts specialized in portal hypertension have different opinions. Some investigators have suggested that patients with a history of variceal bleeding could receive either β-blockers or EVL to prevent rebleeding, whereas the combination of EVL and nadolol could be reserved for patients failed in EVL or β-blocker alone.[8,97] On the other hand, others suggest that a β-blocker should be combined with EVL as the treatment of choice to prevent recurrent variceal hemorrhage.[98] Moreover, β-blockers should be employed during the course of EVL as well as after variceal obliteration to prevent variceal recurrence. It has been shown that if patients on drug therapy could reduce the hepatic venous pressure gradient (HVPG) by more than 20% of basal value or HVPG was lowered to less than 12 mm Hg, the rebleeding rate could be significantly reduced.[8] As a result, if patients receiving medical therapy could achieve an ideal HVPG, combination of endoscopic therapy would be obviated. However, HVPG cannot be routinely performed in clinical practice. Furthermore, some patients may die of variceal hemorrhage if rebleeding episodes cannot be easily controlled. Hence, combination of medical and endoscopic therapy is the favored treatment of choice in the prevention of variceal rebleeding, provided that patients do not have contraindications to either therapy.

RESCUE THERAPY FOR ENDOSCOPIC TREATMENT FAILURE

After repeated endoscopic therapies or combination of endoscopic and pharmacologic therapy, approximately 20% of patients may still encounter rebleeding.

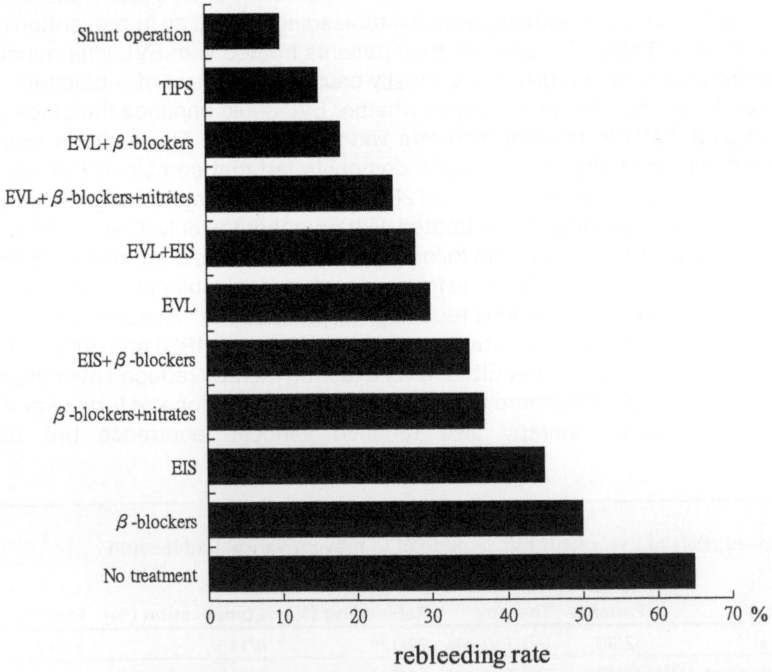

Fig. 1. Relative effectiveness of various modalities in the prevention of variceal rebleeding. The figures of rebleeding rates are estimates of rebleeding within 2 years of treatment based on available meta-analyses and/or publications.

Alternative methods are required to rescue these patients. Liver transplantation may be considered if patients are good candidates and donor livers are available. If liver transplantation is not feasible, shunt operation may be considered for patients with good liver reserve, and TIPS may be considered for patients with poor liver reserve.[99–102] Several studies have compared the efficacy and safety of TIPS with endoscopic therapy in the prevention of variceal rebleeding.[103,104] Meta-analyses disclosed that variceal rebleeding was significantly more frequent with endoscopic therapy (47%) compared with TIPS (19%).[105] The survival was similar between both therapies, but TIPS is associated with a significantly higher incidence of hepatic encephalopathy. Based on these observations, TIPS is not favored as a first-line therapy for prevention of variceal rebleeding but rather as a rescue therapy for endoscopic and pharmacologic treatment failure.[106,107]

SUMMARY

Over the past 30 years, endoscopic therapy has become widely accepted for the prevention of esophageal variceal rebleeding. There are several endoscopic methods for the clinician to choose from. EVL has replaced EIS as the treatment of choice for the prevention of variceal rebleeding. The efficacy of EVL alone is at least as effective as medical therapy in the reduction of variceal rebleeding, but may be associated with

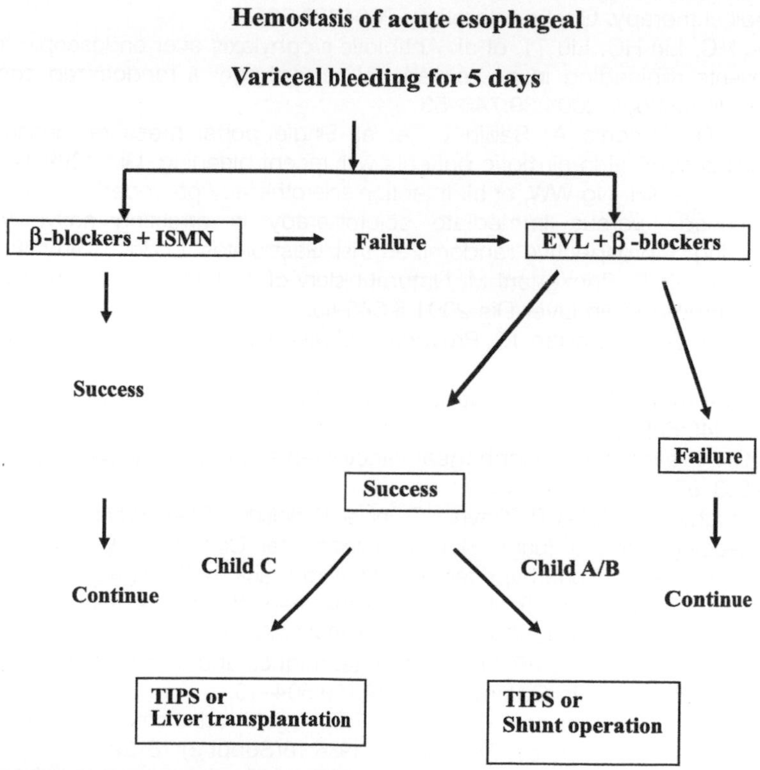

Fig. 2. Algorithm for prevention of esophageal variceal rebleeding. EVL, endoscopic variceal ligation; ISMN, isosorbide mononitrate; TIPS, transjugular intrahepatic portosystemic stent shunt.

more complications. In patients who are intolerant or have contraindications to β-blockers, EVL alone can be employed as the first-line treatment. Regular surveillance at intervals of 3 to 6 months is advised for patients achieving variceal obliteration by endoscopic therapy. On variceal obliteration achieved by EVL, EIS with low-dose sclerosants or argon plasma could be applied to prevent variceal recurrence. Synchronous combination of EVL and EIS does not confer benefit than either therapy alone. A combined approach with EVL and nadolol can be used as a first-line treatment or be reserved until pharmacologic or endoscopic therapy failure. Shunt operation and TIPS are recommended to be reserved for esophageal varices that cannot be managed by endoscopic and pharmacologic modalities. If patients belong to Child class C with repeated variceal bleeding, they probably are better to be on the waiting list for liver transplantation. The comparison of approximate rebleeding rates with various modalities within 2 years is shown in **Fig. 1**. The algorithm for the prevention of esophageal variceal hemorrhage is shown in **Fig. 2**.

REFERENCES

1. Graham DY, Smith JL. The course of patients after variceal hemorrhage. Gastroenterology 1981;80:800–9.
2. D'Amico G, de Franchis R. Upper digestive bleeding in cirrhosis. Post-therapeutic outcome and prognostic indicators. Hepatology 2003;38:599–612.
3. Mihas AA, Sanyal AJ. Recurrent variceal bleeding despite endoscopic and medical therapy. Gastroenterology 2004;127:621–9.
4. Hou MC, Lin HC, Liu TT, et al. Antibiotic prophylaxis after endoscopic therapy prevents rebleeding in acute variceal hemorrhage: a randomized controlled trial. Hepatology 2004;39:746–53.
5. Patch D, Armonis A, Sabin C, et al. Single portal pressure measurement predicts survival in cirrhotic patients with recent bleeding. Gut 1999;44:264–9.
6. Lo GH, Lai KH, Ng WW, et al. Injection sclerotherapy preceded by esophageal tamponade versus immediate sclerotherapy in arresting active variceal bleeding: a prospective randomized trial. Gastrointest Endosc 1992;38:421–4.
7. de Franchis R, Primignani M. Natural history of portal hypertension in patients with cirrhosis. Clin Liver Dis 2001;5:645–63.
8. Bosch J, Garcia-Pagan JC. Prevention of variceal rebleeding. Lancet 2003;361: 952–4.
9. Sharara AI, Rockey DC. Gastroesophageal variceal hemorrhage. N Engl J Med 2001;345:669–81.
10. Lo GH. Prevention of esophageal variceal rebleeding. J Chin Med Assoc 2006; 69:553–60.
11. Burroughs AK, Cales P, Kravetz D, et al. Definition of key events—last attempt? Proceedings of the fourth Baveno International Consensus Workshop. In: de Franchis R, editor. Portal hypertension IV. Oxford: Blackwell Publishing; 2006. p. 11–39.
12. Crafoord C, Frenckner P. New surgical treatment of varicose veins of the esophagus. Acta Otolaryngol (Stockholm) 1939;27:422–9.
13. Sanowski RA, Waring JP. Endoscopic techniques and complications in variceal sclerotherapy. J Clin Gastroenterol 1987;9:504–13.
14. Jensen DM, Machicado GA, Silpa M. Esophageal varix hemorrhage and sclerotherapy—animal studies. Endoscopy 1986;18(Suppl 2):18–22.
15. Westaby D, Melai WM, MacDougall BRD, et al. Injection sclerotherapy for esophageal varices: a prospective, randomized trial of different treatment schedules. Gut 1984;25:129–32.

16. Conn HO. Endoscopic sclerotherapy: an analysis of variants. Hepatology 1983; 3:769–71.
17. Johnston GW, Rodgers HW. A review of 15 years' experience in the use of sclerotherapy in the control of acute hemorrhage from esophageal varices. Br J Surg 1973;60:797–800.
18. Macdougall BR, Westaby D, Theodossi A, et al. Increased long-term survival in variceal hemorrhage using injection sclerotherapy. Results of a controlled trial. Lancet 1982;1:124–7.
19. Terblanche J, Bornman PC, Kahn D, et al. Failure of repeated injection sclerotherapy to improve long-term survival after esophageal variceal bleeding. A five-year prospective controlled clinical trial. Lancet 1983;2(8363): 1328–32.
20. Sclerotherapy after first variceal hemorrhage in cirrhosis. A randomized multicenter trial. The Copenhagen Esophageal Varices Sclerotherapy Project. N Engl J Med 1984;311:1594–600.
21. Korula J, Balart LA, Radvan G, et al. A prospective, randomized and controlled trial of chronic esophageal variceal sclerotherapy. Hepatology 1985;5:584–9.
22. Williams R, Westaby D. Endoscopic sclerotherapy for esophageal varices. Dig Dis Sci 1986;31(Suppl 9):108S–21S.
23. Schuman BM, Beckman JW, Tedesco FJ, et al. Complications of endoscopic injection sclerotherapy: a review. Am J Gastroenterol 1987;82:823–30.
24. Cohen LB, Korsten MA, Scherl EJ, et al. Bacteremia after endoscopic injection sclerosis. Gastrointest Endosc 1983;29:198–200.
25. Sarles HE, Sanowski RA, Talbert G. Course and complications of endoscopic variceal sclerotherapy: a prospective study of 50 patients. Am J Gastroenterol 1985;80:595–9.
26. Haynes WC, Sanowski RA, Foutch PG, et al. Esophageal strictures following endoscopic variceal sclerotherapy: clinical course and response to dilation therapy. Gastrointest Endosc 1986;32:202–5.
27. Soehendra N, Binmoeller KF. Is sclerotherapy out? Endoscopy 1997;29:283–4.
28. de Franchis R, Primignani M. Endoscopic treatments for portal hypertension. Semin Liver Dis 1999;19:439–55.
29. Infante-Rivard C, Esnaola S, Villeneuve JP. Role of endoscopic variceal sclerotherapy in the long- term management of variceal bleeding: a meta-analysis. Gastroenterology 1989;96:1087–92.
30. Lai KH, Chiang TT, Tsai YT, et al. Follow-up study after endoscopic injection sclerotherapy. Chin J Gastroenterol 1985;2:164–70.
31. Kitano S, Koyanagi N, Iso Y, et al. Prevention of recurrence of esophageal varices after endoscopic injection sclerotherapy with ethanolamine oleate. Hepatology 1987;7:810–5.
32. Kitano S, Baatar D. Endoscopic treatment for esophageal varices: will there be a place for sclerotherapy during the forthcoming era of ligation? Gastrointest Endosc 2000;52:226–32.
33. Bernard B, Lebrec D, Mathurin P, et al. Propranolol and sclerotherapy in the prevention of gastrointestinal rebleeding in patients with cirrhosis: a meta-analysis. J Hepatol 1997;26:312–24.
34. Villanueva C, Balanzo J, Novella MT, et al. Nadolol plus isosorbide mononitrate compared with sclerotherapy for the prevention of variceal rebleeding. N Engl J Med 1996;334:1624–9.
35. D'Amico G, Pagliaro L, Bosch J. Pharmacological treatment of portal hypertension: an evidence-based approach. Semin Liver Dis 1999;19:475–505.

36. Stiegmann GV, Goff JS. Endoscopic esophageal varix ligation: preliminary clinical experience. Gastrointest Endosc 1988;34:113–7.
37. Naga MI, Okasha HH, Foda AR. Detachable endoloop vs. band ligation for bleeding esophageal varices. Gastrointest Endosc 2004;59:804–9.
38. Young MF, Sanowski RA, Rasche R. Comparison and characterization of ulceration induced by endoscopic ligation of esophageal varices versus endoscopic sclerotherapy. Gastrointest Endosc 1993;39:119–22.
39. Bolognesi M, Balducci G, Garcia- Tsao, et al. Complications in the medical treatment of portal hypertension. Proceedings of the third Baveno international consensus workshop on definitions, methodology and therapeutic strategies. In: de Franchis R, editor. Portal hypertension III. Oxford (UK): Blackwell Science; 2001. p. 180–201.
40. Stiegmann GV, Goff JS, Michaletz-Onody PA, et al. Endoscopic sclerotherapy as compared with endoscopic ligation for bleeding esophageal varices. N Engl J Med 1992;326:1527–32.
41. Laine L, El-Newihi HM, Migikovsky B, et al. Endoscopic ligation compared with sclerotherapy for the treatment of bleeding esophageal varices. Ann Intern Med 1993;119:1–7.
42. Gimson AES, Ramage JK, Panos MZ, et al. Randomised trial of variceal banding ligation versus injection sclerotherapy for bleeding esophageal varices. Lancet 1993;342:391–4.
43. Lo GH, Lai KH, Cheng JS, et al. A prospective, randomized trial of sclerotherapy versus ligation in the management of bleeding esophageal varices. Hepatology 1995;22:466–71.
44. Laine L, Cook D. Endoscopic ligation compared with sclerotherapy for treatment of esophageal variceal bleeding. Ann Intern Med 1995;121:280–7.
45. Lo GH, Lai KH, Shen MT, et al. A comparison of the incidence of transient bacteremia and infectious sequelae after sclerotherapy and rubber band ligation of bleeding esophageal varices. Gastrointest Endosc 1994;40:675–9.
46. Laine L. Ligation: endoscopic treatment of choice for patients with bleeding esophageal varices? Hepatology 1995;22:663–5.
47. Hou MC, Lin HC, Kuo BIT, et al. Comparison of endoscopic variceal injection sclerotherapy and ligation for the treatment of esophageal variceal hemorrhage: A prospective randomized trial. Hepatology 1995;21:1517–22.
48. Sarin SK, Govil A, Jain AK. Prospective randomized trial of endoscopic sclerotherapy versus variceal band ligation for esophageal varices: influence on gastropathy, gastric varices and variceal recurrence. J Hepatol 1997;26:826–32.
49. Hou MC, Lin HC, Lee FY, et al. Recurrence of esophageal varices following endoscopic treatment and its impact on rebleeding: comparison of sclerotherapy and ligation. J Hepatol 2000;32:202–8.
50. Garcia-Tsao G, Sanyal AJ, Grace ND, et al. Prevention and management of gastroesophageal varices and variceal hemorrhage in cirrhosis. Hepatology 2007;46:922–38.
51. Yoshida H, Mamada Y, Taniai N, et al. A randomized controlled trial of bimonthly versus biweekly endoscopic variceal ligation of esophageal varices. Am J Gastroenterol 2005;100:2005–9.
52. Harewood GC, Baron TH, Song LM. Factors predicting success of endoscopic variceal ligation for secondary prophylaxis of esophageal variceal bleeding. J Gastroenterol Hepatol 2006;21:237–41.

53. Ramirez FC, Colon VJ, Landan D, et al. The effects of the number of rubber bands placed at each endoscopic session upon variceal outcomes: a prospective, randomized study. Am J Gastroenterol 2007;102:1372–6.
54. Viazis N, Armonis A, Vlachogiannakos J, et al. Effects of endoscopic variceal treatment on esophageal function: a prospective, randomized study. Eur J Gastroenterol Hepatol 2002;14:263–9.
55. Chen SM, Lo GH, Lai KH, et al. Influence of endoscopic variceal ligation on esophageal motility. J Gastroenterol Hepatol 1999;14:231–5.
56. Sauerbruch T, Schepke M. Sclerotherapy is out—nearly. Endoscopy 1997;29: 281–2.
57. Villanueva C, Minyana J, Ortiz J, et al. Endoscopic ligation compared with combined treatment with nadolol and isosorbide mononitrate to prevent recurrent variceal rebleeding. N Engl J Med 2001;345:647–55.
58. Lo GH, Chen WC, Chen MH, et al. A prospective, randomized trial of endoscopic variceal ligation versus nadolol and isosorbide mononitrate for the prevention of esophageal variceal rebleeding. Gastroenterology 2002;123:728–34.
59. Patch D, Sabin CA, Goulis J, et al. A randomized, controlled trial of medical therapy versus endoscopic ligation for the prevention of variceal rebleeding in patients with cirrhosis. Gastroenterology 2002;123:1013–9.
60. Romero G, Kravetz D, Argonz J, et al. Nadolol plus isosorbide mononitrate compared with banding plus low volume sclerotherapy for prevention of variceal rebleeding in patients with cirrhosis. Hepatology 2004;40(Suppl 1):204A.
61. Sarin SK, Wadhawan M, Gupta R, et al. Evaluation of endoscopic variceal ligation (EVL) versus propranolol plus isosorbide mononitrate/nadolol (ISMN) in the prevention of variceal rebleeding: comparison of cirrhotic and noncirrhotic patients. Dig Dis Sci 2005;50:1538–47.
62. Garcia-Pagan JC, Bosch J. Endoscopic band ligation in the treatment of portal hypertension. Nat Clin Pract Gastroenterol Hepatol 2005;2:526–35.
63. Lo GH, Chen WC, Lin CK, et al. Improved survival in patients receiving medical therapy as compared with banding ligation for the prevention of esophageal variceal rebleeding. Hepatology 2008;48:580–7.
64. Hayashi T, Yonezawa M, Kuwabara T. The study on stanch clip for the treatment by endoscopy. Gastroenterol Endosc 1975;17:92–101.
65. Hachisu T. Evaluation of endoscopic hemostasis using an improved clipping apparatus. Surg Endosc 1988;2:207–30.
66. Yol S, Belviranli M, Kartal TA. Endoscopic clipping vs. band ligation in the management of bleeding esophageal varices. Surg Endosc 2003;17:38–42.
67. Lo GH, Lai KH, Cheng JS, et al. A prospective, randomized trial of butyl cyanoacrylate injection versus band ligation in the management of bleeding gastric varices. Hepatology 2001;33:1060–4.
68. Feretis C, Dimopoulos C, Benakis P, et al. Endoscopic hemostasis of esophageal and gastric variceal bleeding with histoacryl. Endoscopy 1990;22:282–4.
69. Sung JJY, Yeo W, Suen R, et al. Injection sclerotherapy for variceal bleeding in patients with hepatocellular carcinoma: cyanoacrylate versus sodium tetradecyl sulfate. Gastrointest Endosc 1998;47:235–9.
70. Marvin R, Christopher CT. Tissue adhesives: a review. Tech Gastrointest Endosc 2006;8:33–7.
71. Evrard S, Dumonceau JM, Delhaye M, et al. Endoscopic histoacryl obliteration vs. propranolol in the prevention of esophagogastric variceal rebleeding: a randomized trial. Endoscopy 2003;9:729–35.

72. Lo GH, Lai KH, Cheng JS, et al. Prevalence of paraesophageal varices and gastric varices in patients achieving variceal obliteration by banding ligation and by injection sclerotherapy. Gastrointest Endosc 1999;49:428–36.
73. Singh P, Pooran N, Indaram A, et al. Combined ligation and sclerotherapy versus ligation alone for secondary prophylaxis of esophageal variceal bleeding: a meta-analysis. Am J Gastroenterol 2002;97:623–9.
74. Hou MC, Chen WC, Lin HC, et al. A new "sandwich" method of combined endoscopic variceal ligation and sclerotherapy versus ligation alone in the treatment of esophageal variceal bleeding: a randomized trial. Gastrointest Endosc 2001;53:572–8.
75. Umehara M, Onda M, Tajiri T, et al. Sclerotherapy plus ligation versus ligation for the treatment of esophageal varices: a prospective randomized study. Gastrointest Endosc 1999;50:7–12.
76. Lo GH, Lai KH, Cheng JS, et al. The additive effect of sclerotherapy to patients receiving repeated endoscopic variceal ligation: a prospective, randomized trial. Hepatology 1998;28:391–5.
77. Cheng YS, Pan S, Lien GS, et al. Adjuvant sclerotherapy after ligation for the treatment of esophageal varices: a prospective, randomized long-term study. Gastrointest Endosc 2001;53:566–71.
78. Garg PK, Joshi YK, Tandon RK. Comparison of endoscopic variceal sclerotherapy with sequential endoscopic band ligation plus low-dose sclerotherapy for secondary prophylaxis of variceal hemorrhage: a prospective randomized study. Gastrointest Endosc 1999;50:369–73.
79. Hashizume M, Ohta M, Kawanaka H, et al. Recurrence rate of esophageal varices with endoscopic banding ligation followed by injection sclerotherapy [letter]. Lancet 1994;344:1643.
80. Monici LT, Meirelles-Santos JO, Soares EC, et al. Microwave coagulation versus sclerotherapy after band ligation to prevent recurrence of high risk of esophageal varices in Child-Pugh's A and B patients. J Gastroenterol 2010;45:204–10.
81. Cipolletta L, Bianco MA, Rotondano G, et al. Endoscopic blockade to prevent resurfacing of esophageal varices. Gastroenterology 2003;124:1545–55.
82. Marrero JA, Scheiman JM. Prevention of recurrent variceal bleeding: as easy as A.P.C. Gastrointest Endosc 2002;56:600–3.
83. Chen WC, Lo GH, Tsai WL, et al. Emergency endoscopic variceal ligation versus somatostatin for acute esophageal variceal bleeding. J Chin Med Assoc 2006; 69:60–7.
84. Hou MC, Lin HC, Chen CH, et al. Changes in portal hypertensive gastropathy after endoscopic variceal sclerotherapy or ligation: an endoscopic observation. Gastrointest Endosc 1995;42:139–44.
85. Lo GH, Lai KH, Cheng JS, et al. The effects of endoscopic variceal ligation and propranolol on portal hypertensive gastropathy: a prospective, controlled trial. Gastrointest Endosc 2001;53:579–84.
86. Sarin SK, Lahoti D, Saxena SP, et al. Prevalence, classification and natural history of gastric varices: a longterm follow-up study in 568 portal hypertension patients. Hepatology 1992;16:1343–9.
87. Korula J, Ralls P. The effect of chronic endoscopic sclerotherapy on portal pressure in cirrhotics. Gastroenterology 1991;101:800–5.
88. Lo GH, Liang HL, Lai KH, et al. The impact of endoscopic variceal ligation on the pressure of the portal venous system. J Hepatol 1996;24:74–80.
89. Lo GH, Lai KH, Lee SD, et al. Does propranolol maintain post-sclerotherapy variceal obliteration? A prospective randomized study. J Gastroenterol Hepatol 1993;8:358–62.

90. Ink O, Martin T, Poynard T, et al. Does elective sclerotherapy improve the efficacy of long-term propranolol for prevention of recurrent bleeding in patients with severe cirrhosis? A prospective multicenter, randomized trial. Hepatology 1992;16:912–9.
91. de Franchis R, Primignani M. Endoscopic treatments for portal hypertension. Sem Liver Dis 1999;19:439–55.
92. Lo GH, Lai KH, Cheng JS, et al. Endoscopic variceal ligation plus nadolol and sucralfate compared with ligation alone for the prevention of variceal rebleeding: a prospective, randomized trial. Hepatology 2000;32:461–5.
93. De la Pena J, Brullet E, Sanchez-Hernandez E, et al. Variceal ligation plus nadolol compared with ligation for prophylaxis of variceal rebleeding: a multicenter trial. Hepatology 2005;41:572–8.
94. Lo GH, Chen WC, Chen MH, et al. A randomized, controlled trial of banding ligation plus drug therapy vs drug therapy alone in the prevention of esophageal variceal rebleeding. J Gastroenterol Hepatol 2009;24:982–7.
95. Garcia-Pagan JC, Villaneuva C, Albillos A, et al. Nadolol plus isosorbide mononitrate alone or associated with band ligation in the prevention of recurrent bleeding: A multicenter randomized controlled trial. Gut 2009;58:1144–50.
96. Gonzalez R, Zamora J, Gomez-Camarero J, et al. Meta-analysis: Combination endoscopic and drug therapy to prevent variceal rebleeding in cirrhosis. Ann Intern Med 2008;15(149):109–22.
97. Garcia-Tsao G. Current management of the complications of cirrhosis and portal hypertension: variceal hemorrhage, ascites, and spontaneous bacterial peritonitis. Gastroenterology 2001;120:726–48.
98. Boyer TD. Pharmacologic treatment of portal hypertension: past, present, and future. Hepatology 2001;34:834–9.
99. Henderson JM. Role of distal splenorenal shunt for long-term management of variceal bleeding. World J Surg 1994;18:205–10.
100. Chau TN, Patch D, Chan YW, et al. "Salvage" transjugular intrahepatic portosystemic shunts: gastric fundal compared with esophageal variceal bleeding. Gastroenterology 1998;114:981–7.
101. Le Moine O, Deviere J, Ghysels M, et al. Transjugular intrahepatic portosystemic shunt as a rescue treatment after sclerotherapy failure in variceal bleeding. Scand J Gastroenterol Suppl 1994;207:23–8.
102. Yang CF, Tzeng WS, Chang JM, et al. Experience with transjugular intrahepatic portosystemic shunts for gastroesophageal variceal bleeding. J Chin Med Assoc 1996;57:204–13.
103. Sauer P, Hansmann J, Richter GM, et al. Endoscopic variceal ligation plus propranolol vs. transjugular intrahepatic portosystemic stent shunt: a long-term randomized trial. Endoscopy 2002;34:690–7.
104. Sanyal AJ, Freedman AM, Luketic VA, et al. Transjugular intrahepatic portosystemic stent shunt compared with endoscopic therapy for the prevention of recurrent variceal hemorrhage: a randomized, controlled trial. Ann Intern Med 1997; 126:849–57.
105. Papatheodoridis G, Goulis J, Leandro G, et al. Transjugular intrahepatic portosystemic shunt compared with endoscopic treatment for prevention of variceal rebleeding: a meta-analysis. Hepatology 1999;30:612–22.
106. Boyer TD, Haskal ZJ. The role of transjugular intrahepatic portosystemic shunt in the management of portal hypertension. Hepatology 2005;41:386–400.
107. Krige JEJ, Shaw JM, Bornman PC. The evolving role of endoscopic treatment for bleeding esophageal varices. World J Surg 2005;29:966–73.

Endoscopic Ultrasound and Fine-needle Aspiration for the Diagnosis of Hepatocellular Carcinoma

Anurag Maheshwari, MD, Sergey Kantsevoy, MD, PhD,
Sanjay Jagannath, MD, Paul J. Thuluvath, MD, FRCP*

KEYWORDS

- Hepatocellular cancer • Surveillance • Endoscopic ultrasound
- Fine-needle aspiration

Hepatocellular cancer (HCC) is the sixth most common cancer in the world with an estimated incidence of more than 650,000 cases per year. The major risk factor associated with the development of HCC is cirrhosis caused by viral hepatitis B or C and chronic alcohol consumption. The overall prognosis of patients with HCC remains poor with 5-year survival estimates that range between 0% and 10%. This dismal prognosis is mainly the result of the advanced stage of HCC at presentation and the background cirrhosis. When diagnosed early, the prognosis for HCC is better with a 5-year disease-free survival rate ranging from 50% after surgical resection or the use of local ablative treatments, to 70% to 80% after liver transplantation. Curative local ablative treatments that have been studied include radiofrequency ablation and percutaneous ethanol injection. Transarterial chemo-embolization also may improve survival significantly. Systematic screening of high-risk patients is key to an early diagnosis of HCC allowing for the use of an appropriate treatment modality.[1] The currently available tools for the screening, surveillance, and diagnosis of HCC in the presence of cirrhosis remain suboptimal. Advancements in treatment in the past 10 years, however, have made HCC a potentially curable disease in a selected group of patients, increasing the impetus to develop effective diagnostic modalities.

Center for Liver and Biliary Diseases, Institute for Digestive Health and Liver Disease, Mercy Medical Center, 301 St Paul Place, Baltimore, MD 21202-2165, USA
* Corresponding author.
E-mail address: thuluvath@gmail.com

Clin Liver Dis 14 (2010) 325–332
doi:10.1016/j.cld.2010.03.014
liver.theclinics.com

This article briefly reviews the current guidelines for surveillance and diagnosis of HCC in high-risk patients and the potential role of endoscopic ultrasound (EUS) and fine-needle aspiration (FNA) for the diagnosis of small HCC.

SURVEILLANCE OF HCC

Surveillance for HCC is cost-effective only when performed in high-risk patients, which includes all patients with cirrhosis. In addition, all patients with hepatitis B irrespective of the presence of cirrhosis are also at a high risk for the development of HCC. Of the populations infected with hepatitis B, the groups considered at highest risk for HCC include Asian men older than 40 years, Asian women older than 50 years, all Africans more than 20 years of age, those with a family history of HCC, and those with high levels of viral replication (high HBV DNA).[1]

HCC surveillance is usually done by radiological imaging as the currently available laboratory tests have inadequate sensitivity or specificity. Laboratory tests that are currently available for clinical use include α-fetoprotein (AFP), des-γ-carboxy-prothrombin, AFP-L3 fraction, α-fucosidase, and glypican 3. AFP is widely used, but lacks adequate sensitivity and specificity. Although a higher cut-off value (>400 ng/mL) may improve the specificity of AFP testing, it reduces its sensitivity to less than 20% making the test of borderline usefulness. Lower cut-off values (>20 ng/mL) may improve the sensitivity (~60%) but reduce the specificity to less than 20%. An increased AFP level (>200 ng/mL) in the presence of a mass on imaging, or an increasing AFP level has a high positive predictive value for the diagnosis of HCC. Despite its limitations, AFP is still used in many centers as a complementary test for surveillance and diagnosis of HCC. Other blood tests such as des-γ-carboxy-prothrombin, AFP-L3 fraction, α-fucosidase, glypican 3, and so forth., have not been adequately tested for screening, surveillance, or diagnosis of HCC.

Most centers depend on imaging modalities such as transabdominal ultrasound (US), computerized tomography (CT), or magnetic resonance imaging (MRI) for surveillance/screening and diagnosis of HCC. Of these modalities, US imaging every 6 to 12 months has been extensively evaluated and noted to have adequate sensitivity (60%–80%) and specificity (~80%), and found to be a cost-effective screening tool. It is currently recommended as one of the tests acceptable for screening high-risk patients for HCC in the guidelines published by the American Association for Study of Liver Disease.[1] This experience, however, is not shared by many hepatologists in the United States, including the authors, for many reasons. US imaging is operator dependent with a variable sensitivity and specificity in the presence of background cirrhosis and obesity. HCC may appear as hyper-, hypo- or isoechoic lesions on US making the diagnosis difficult in the presence of underlying cirrhosis with concomitant regenerating or dysplastic nodules. Moreover, the overall sensitivity is only around 20% for tumors less than 1 cm. Although not well studied as a surveillance/screening test, because of its diagnostic superiority, most centers in the United States use a triple-phase high-resolution CT scan or contrast-enhanced MRI as their test of choice for screening of HCC. With improved technology, the sensitivity of CT and MRI imaging has significantly increased and the specificity has decreased. A firm diagnosis of HCC is currently established if a mass lesion shows early wash-out on the triple-phase CT scan, or 2 separate imaging modalities are suggestive of HCC, or a combination of one imaging test suggestive of HCC associated with concomitant increase of AFP (≥200 ng/mL) levels. In the absence of these criteria, histology is the only firm method of confirming the diagnosis of HCC. The ability to obtain a biopsy becomes difficult when small lesions, identified on CT or MRI, are not readily visualized on transabdominal US, which happens frequently in our experience. Although a biopsy of some of these lesions could be obtained under CT guidance, this requires expertise that is not available at all centers. Therefore, investigators are in search of better laboratory tests (including biomarkers) and imaging modalities for screening and diagnosis of HCC. There have been a few preliminary studies that have suggested a role for EUS/FNA in the diagnosis of HCC.

ROLE OF EUS AND FNA

EUS combines endoscopy and ultrasound to obtain images and information about the digestive tract and the surrounding tissue and organs. Because of its close proximity to the surrounding organs, the resultant US images are often more accurate and detailed than those obtained by traditional US imaging (**Fig. 1**). EUS is an accepted diagnostic mode for staging of certain cancers (esophagus, stomach, pancreas, rectum, and lung), for the evaluation of chronic pancreatitis, pancreatic masses or cysts, and submucosal lesions in the gastrointestinal tract. EUS-guided FNA has emerged as a key adjunct to standard endosonography that allows the tissue diagnosis of submucosal lesions, extraluminal lesions, and sampling of lymph nodes. The current clinical usefulness of EUS and EUS-FNA seems to be greatest for the diagnosis and staging of pancreatic cancer and for the staging of malignant tumors of the esophagus.

Experience with EUS-FNA in the last decade has found it to be a reliable tool for the evaluation of a host of intrathoracic and intra-abdominal lesions with less emphasis on examination of liver lesions. More recently, many investigators have reported their EUS-FNA experience for tissue diagnosis of liver lesions (**Fig. 2**). A prospective study by Nguyen and colleagues[2] evaluated the liver by EUS $\pm$ FNA in 574 patients with

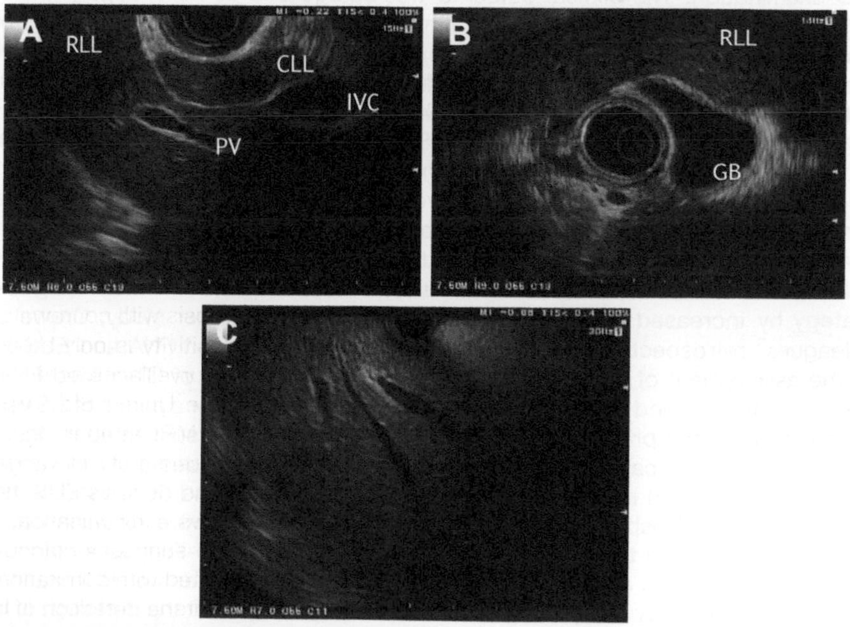

Fig. 1. (*A, B*) EUS appearance of liver and vasculature. CLL, caudate lobe of liver; GB, gall bladder; IVC, inferior vena cava; PV, portal vein; RLL, right lobe of liver. (*C*) Hepatic veins.

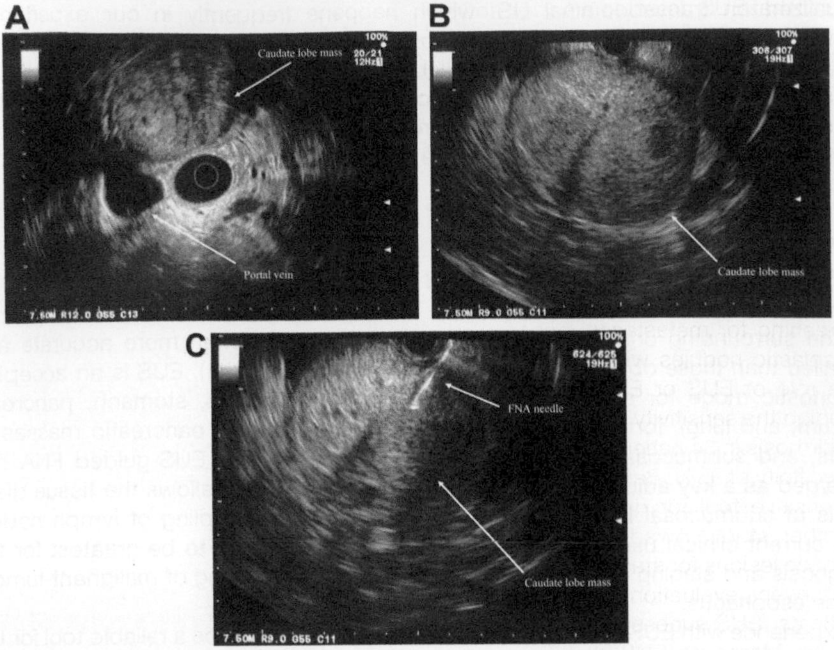

Fig. 2. EUS appearances of a caudate lobe liver mass (*A* and *B*) and EUS guided fine needle aspiration (FNA) (*C*).

a history or suspicion of gastrointestinal or pulmonary malignancy who underwent EUS examination. The clinical outcome was categorized as no change (results of EUS-FNA made no difference in clinical management), avoided surgery (results prevented unnecessary surgical intervention), upstaged tumor (results led to upstaging of primary malignant tumor), or made a firm diagnosis (results led to a diagnosis of malignant tumor). In this study, 14 (2.4%) patients were found to have focal liver lesions and these patients underwent EUS-FNA. A total of 15 liver lesions were aspirated, 14 were malignant and 1 was benign. Previous CT imaging had shown liver lesions in only 3 of 14 (21%) patients. Seven of 14 patients had a known cancer diagnosis and for the other 7, the initial diagnosis of cancer was made by means of EUS-FNA of the liver lesions. This study concluded that EUS examination was able to detect small focal liver lesions not found on CT, and EUS-FNA may change the management strategy by increased accuracy of cancer staging.[2] In another study, Crowe and colleagues[3] retrospectively compared the results of CT-guided FNA and EUS-FNA for the assessment of liver lesions, and described the results of CT-guided FNA of 34 patients for a period of 6 years and EUS-FNA of 16 patients for a period of 2.5 years. In both groups, the primary indication for FNA sampling was suspected metastatic cancer (CT, 41% of cases vs EUS, 56%). Both techniques yielded a similar range of benign, atypical, and malignant diagnoses (CT 26%, 18%, and 56% vs EUS 19%, 25%, and 56%). Despite the major limitations of a retrospective examination, the investigators claimed that EUS-FNA was comparable with CT-FNA as a diagnostic test for the evaluation of hepatic lesions, but there were some anatomic limitations.

A more recent study compared the efficacy of EUS and CT for the detection of liver metastases in 132 patients with newly diagnosed upper gastrointestinal or lung cancer and found a diagnostic accuracy of 98% with EUS and 92% with CT scan.[4] The study found that EUS detected a significantly higher number of liver lesions than CT scan (40 vs 19, $P<.05$). In addition, CT imaging classified 8 cases as being too small to be characterized, and of these, EUS-FNA was able to correctly classify these lesions in 7 cases (3/3 malignant and 4/5 benign lesions). This study did not report any complications as a result of EUS-FNA. The major limitation of the study was that the endosonographer was not blinded to the results of the CT imaging. In addition, although only one experienced endoscopist performed all EUS, the CT imaging was interpreted by multiple radiologists. The variable experiences of the radiologists and the previous knowledge of CT findings may have skewed the results in favor of the endosonographer.

EUS imaging of the liver for HCC screening or surveillance is different from that of screening for metastases, because HCC frequently coexists with regenerative and dysplastic nodules with background cirrhosis. There is only limited information on the role of EUS or EUS-FNA in the presence of cirrhosis. Dodd and colleagues[5] studied the sensitivity and specificity of EUS for the diagnosis of HCC in the presence of cirrhosis in 34 patients and found a sensitivity of 50% (lesion sensitivity of 45%) and specificity of 98%. Based on their study, the investigators concluded that EUS was an insensitive tool for detection of malignant lesions in end-stage cirrhotic livers. In another study, Awad and colleagues[6] conducted the preoperative evaluation of hepatic lesions for staging of HCC and liver metastases in 14 patients. These patients underwent evaluation with conventional dynamic CT imaging and EUS. In all 14 patients, EUS successfully identified hepatic lesions ranging in size from 0.3 cm to 14 cm. Moreover, EUS identified new or additional lesions in 28% (4/14 patients), all less than 0.5 cm in size; these findings influenced the clinical management of these patients. In 2/14 patients EUS correctly identified liver lesions described as suspicious by CT scan to be hemangiomas. Nine patients underwent EUS-guided FNA of hepatic lesions and all FNA passes yielded adequate specimens. The investigators suggested that EUS was a feasible preoperative staging tool for suspicious liver masses on CT scan, and EUS could detect smaller hepatic lesions missed by dynamic CT scans. They concluded that EUS-FNA could play an important role in staging and clinical management decisions. In addition to these case series, 2 case reports have been published where EUS-FNA was reliably used to diagnose metastatic HCC in patients with portal vein thrombosis.[7,8]

A more recent, prospective study compared the accuracy of EUS with CT for the detection of primary liver tumors in 17 high-risk patients with abnormal imaging and increased AFP levels.[9] Eight of 17 patients in the study had HCC and 1 had cholangiocarcinoma; EUS-FNA established the diagnosis in 7 of the 8 patients with HCC. The diagnostic accuracies of US, CT, MRI, and EUS-FNA were 38%, 69%, 92%, and 94%, respectively. Although these differences were not statistically significant, the combined accuracy of EUS with FNA showed a superior trend. In this study, the smallest lesion visualized by EUS and confirmed by FNA cytology was 4 mm in size. Current experience suggests that the diagnosis of HCC is highly dependent on the size of the lesion, with tumors less than 2 cm in size being difficult to image and even more difficult to biopsy. If the reported claims of higher sensitivity of EUS for the detection of smaller HCC lesions are confirmed by larger studies, EUS would have superiority over conventional CT imaging. The ability to perform imaging and tissue sampling in a single session and the ability to sample subcentimeter lesions is a distinct advantage over US, CT, and MRI imaging.

There has been more interest in advancing these techniques further. A recent report described the use of elastography in conjunction with EUS imaging to characterize liver lesions based on the relative stiffness of the tissue within the liver lesion

6. Awad SS, Fagan S, Abudayyeh S, et al. Preoperative evaluation of hepatic lesions for the staging of hepatocellular and metastatic liver carcinoma using endoscopic ultrasonography. Am J Surg 2002;184(6):601–4.
7. Storch I, Gomez C, Contreras F, et al. Hepatocellular carcinoma (HCC) with portal vein invasion, masquerading as pancreatic mass, diagnosed by endoscopic ultrasound-guided fine needle aspiration (EUS-FNA). Dig Dis Sci 2007;52(3):789–91.
8. Lai R, Stephens V, Bardales R. Diagnosis and staging of hepatocellular carcinoma by EUS-FNA of a portal vein thrombus. Gastrointest Endosc 2004;59(4):574–7.
9. Singh P, Erickson RA, Mukhopadhyay P, et al. EUS for detection of the hepatocellular carcinoma: results of a prospective study. Gastrointest Endosc 2007;66(2):265–73.
10. Rustemovic N, Hrstic I, Opacic M, et al. EUS elastography in the diagnosis of focal liver lesions. Gastrointest Endosc 2007;66(4):823–4.
11. Thuluvath PJ. EUS-guided FNA could be another important tool for the early diagnosis of hepatocellular carcinoma. Gastrointest Endosc 2007;66(2):274–6.
12. Al-Haddad M, Wallace MB, Woodward TA, et al. The safety of fine-needle aspiration guided by endoscopic ultrasound: a prospective study. Endoscopy 2008;40(3):204–8.
13. Eloubeidi MA, Tamhane A, Varadarajulu S, et al. Frequency of major complications after EUS-guided FNA of solid pancreatic masses: a prospective evaluation. Gastrointest Endosc 2006;63(4):622–9.
14. Eloubeidi MA, Chen VK, Eltoum IA, et al. Endoscopic ultrasound-guided fine needle aspiration biopsy of patients with suspected pancreatic cancer: diagnostic accuracy and acute and 30-day complications. Am J Gastroenterol 2003;98(12):2663–8.

Endoscopic Retrograde Cholangiopancreatography in the Diagnosis and Management of Cholangiocarcinoma

Nayantara Coelho-Prabhu, MD, Todd H. Baron, MD*

KEYWORDS

- Cholangiocarcinoma
- Endoscopic retrograde cholangiopancreatography
- Diagnosis • Management

Cholangiocarcinomas (CCAs) are rare malignancies that arise from the biliary epithelium. CCAs are classified based on location into intrahepatic, perihilar, and distal CCAs.[1] Perihilar tumors (also called Klatskin tumors) are the commonest type, accounting for about 60% to 80% of all CCAs seen at tertiary hospitals while distal extrahepatic cancers are the next most common at 20% to 30%. Intrahepatic tumors are those that arise within the liver and comprise about 10%. Extrahepatic tumors can be further described as mass-forming (nodular), periductal infiltrating (sclerosing), or intraductal (papillary),[2] and this classification correlates with the morphology of the tumor. The prognosis of CCA is poor because most tumors are detected late in their course after metastases have developed. Detection is late because most of these cancers grow longitudinally along the duct and hence only become symptomatic when a larger tumor burden is present. Surgery is the definitive treatment for CCA[3]; however, only a minority of patients are candidates. Palliative therapy is more common, and is discussed later in this article.

Risk factors for development of CCA include increasing age, primary sclerosing cholangitis (PSC), ulcerative colitis, choledochal cysts, Caroli disease, intrahepatic stones, choledocholithiasis, infection with parasites such as *Clonorchis sinensis*,[4] and exposure to Thorotrast.

This work was not supported by any grants.
The authors have no financial disclosures or conflicts to declare.
Division of Gastroenterology and Hepatology, Mayo Clinic Rochester, 200 First Street SW, Rochester, MN 55905, USA
* Corresponding author.
E-mail address: baron.todd@mayo.edu

Clin Liver Dis 14 (2010) 333–348
doi:10.1016/j.cld.2010.03.011

Intrahepatic CCAs usually present as mass lesions that are asymptomatic or cause nonspecific systemic symptoms such as fatigue, fever, and weight loss. Hilar and extrahepatic tumors most commonly present with jaundice, though cholangitis also can be seen. Tumor markers such as carbohydrate antigen 19-9 and carcinoembryonic antigen have been used to diagnose CCA, but these are nonspecific and may be elevated in infection, inflammation, or any obstruction.

Endoscopic retrograde cholangiopancreatography (ERCP) has been used for the diagnosis and management of CCA for many years. In this review, the authors summarize the data regarding the application of ERCP in the diagnosis and management of CCA.

DIAGNOSIS

Ultrasonography is often the first imaging test obtained in patients who present with jaundice. Ultrasonography can identify duct dilation,[5] which may be seen with hilar or distal bile duct tumors but does not allow a definitive diagnosis to be made. Computed tomography (CT) with contrast can determine the extent of the lesion, its location, and presence of hepatic atrophy and metastases. Magnetic resonance imaging (MRI) with magnetic resonance cholangiopancreatography (MRCP) is the radiologic imaging of choice for patients with suspected CCA.[6,7] These modalities allow identification of local tumor extension, enlarged lymph nodes, and metastases. MRI also allows the liver parenchyma to be characterized. MRI is especially useful in patients with total biliary obstruction, and can identify the proximal and distal extent of the tumor. Endoscopic ultrasound (EUS) can be used to identify hilar lesions and lymph nodes[8]; it can also be used to confirm the diagnosis by aspiration with a sensitivity of 75% to 89% for biliary strictures.[9–11]

ERCP allows tissue acquisition for cytologic and histologic analysis while also delineating the tumor and the rest of the biliary tree. Cholangiographic features suggestive of malignancy include stricture length greater than 10 mm, irregular margins, and an abrupt transition from normal duct to stricture, also called shouldering (**Fig. 1**).[12] However, this only suggests a malignancy, and a definitive diagnosis can only be made with tissue histology. Tissue can be obtained by using a cytology brush, or by biopsy or bile aspiration, or a combination of these techniques. Biopsies can also be obtained under direct vision using per-oral cholangioscopy.

ERCP brush cytology has a sensitivity of 30% to 50% and specificity approaching 100% for detection of CCA (**Fig. 2**A).[13–17] In an attempt to improve the sensitivity, bile aspiration for cytologic evaluation and cytologic sampling of tissue from removed stents has been studied. However, these methods have not been shown to greatly increase the diagnostic yield.[18] Another strategy employed to improve the diagnostic yield of cytology is stricture dilation followed by brush cytology. De Bellis and colleagues[19] performed a prospective study comparing cytologic yield before and after stricture dilation. No increase in sensitivity was seen, though the combined yield of brush cytology taken before and after increased the cancer detection rate from 33% to 44% (P<.01). This result suggests that obtaining more tissue samples increases the sensitivity of brush cytology. Fogel and colleagues[20] performed a prospective randomized study comparing the use of a standard cytology brush with a longer brush, and found that despite improved cellularity in the specimens, the cancer detection rate was unchanged. Mansfield and colleagues[16] used a screw stent retriever to acquire tissue and compared the findings with those taken with a standard cytology brush. The latter was superior in terms of cancer detection. Brush cytology is the simplest and safest technique of tissue collection, with only one complication ever

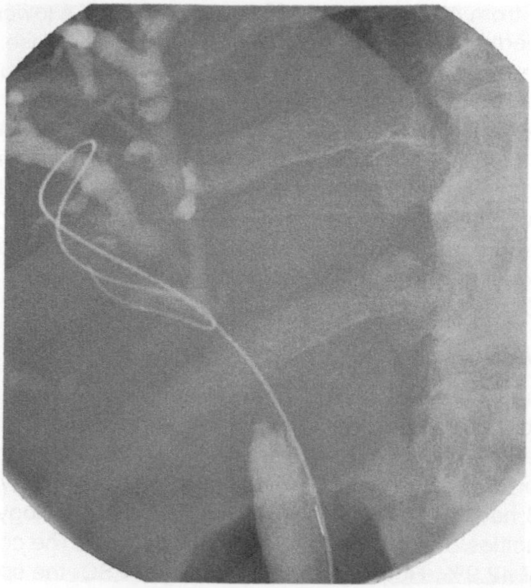

Fig. 1. Cholangiogram showing hilar stricture with shouldering and dilated proximal biliary ductal system.

reported.[21] However, if this is the only sampling modality used, it may be best to obtain multiple samples to maximize diagnostic yield.

In a 2008 study, Dumonceau and colleagues[22] compared the use of a basket and a standard biliary brush, and found that the sensitivity increased from 48% in the brush group to 80% in the basket group, and this was further increased by stricture dilation. Transpapillary biopsies taken under fluoroscopic guidance have a sensitivity of 40% to 80% for detection of bile duct tumors, but the yield is highly dependent on the experience of the endoscopist and the amount of tissue obtained during the biopsy.[14,23,24] Substantial data support the use of performing multiple sampling techniques during ERCP to enhance diagnostic yield.[25] The combined yield of brush and biopsy

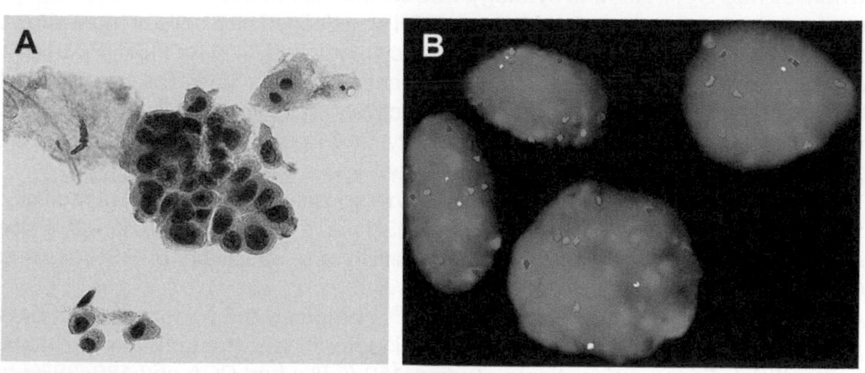

Fig. 2. (*A*) Routine cytology from bile duct brushings of a cholangiocarcinoma showing high nuclear to cytoplasmic ratio and prominent nucleoli. (*B*) FISH from bile duct brushings of a cholangiocarcinoma showing polysomy in the cells.

increases the yield from 40% up to 70%[26] though the yield is lower for hilar CCAs.[27] Intraductal fine-needle aspiration does not appear to increase the yield unless combined with other modalities.[14,28] In the authors' institution, both transpapillary biopsy and brushing are routinely performed.

Chromosomal instability is nearly universal in cancerous cells and results in aneuploidy (abnormalities in the number of chromosomes within a cell) and/or structural chromosomal changes (gene deletion or amplification). It is known that 80% of biliary cancers exhibit aneuploidy.[29] Hence, in addition to routine cytology and pathology, newer cytologic techniques can be recommended to diagnose aneuploidy. These methods include digital image analysis (DIA) and fluorescent in situ hybridization (FISH) (see **Fig. 2**B).

Digital Image Analysis

DIA allows for quantification of DNA content (aneuploidy or tetraploidy) in individual cells using spectrophotometric principles.[30] Therefore it is useful when the sample obtained has limited cellularity. In a study published in 2004 from the authors' institution,[31] DIA was compared with routine cytology in 100 patients with bile duct strictures, of whom 33 had CCA. The sensitivities of DIA and cytology were 39.3% and 17.9% with specificities of 77.3% and 97.7%, respectively. The combination of both had a sensitivity of 42.9%. However, for patients with PSC, the specificity was even lower. Moreno-Luna and colleagues[32] studied the added advantage of DIA and FISH when cytology was negative, and found that DIA added little to the diagnosis but FISH increased the sensitivity to 35% to 60%.

In a more recent prospective study[33] in which intraductal ultrasound, cytology, DIA, and FISH were compared in 86 patients with indeterminate strictures, DIA had a sensitivity of 38% with specificity of 95%. For patients with PSC, the sensitivity dropped to 21%. However, a recent study by Fritcher and colleagues[34] compared the performance of brushings obtained during ERCP in patients with indeterminate strictures using cytology, DIA, and FISH. By multivariate statistical analysis DIA was not an independent predictor of malignancy, and therefore this test is no longer performed.

Fluorescence In Situ Hybridization

FISH uses fluorescently labeled DNA probes to detect chromosomal abnormalities, particularly abnormal loss or gain of chromosomes. FISH assesses chromosomes 3, 7, 17, and 9p21. Kipp and colleagues[35] studied 133 patients with biliary strictures, of whom 39 had CCA. Routine cytology was compared with FISH using brush samples and bile aspiration samples. Positivity on FISH was defined as 5 cells or more showing polysomy. The sensitivity was 15% for brush cytology and 34% for FISH ($P<.01$) while combined sensitivity of FISH for aspirate and brushings was 35%. The specificities for cytology and FISH were 98% and 91%, respectively. Thus, the sensitivity for FISH was better but at the expense of a lower specificity. Of 71 patients with PSC, 16 had CCA with a slightly higher sensitivity and specificity.

The presence of trisomy 7 alone on FISH had a sensitivity of 64% with a specificity of 82%. However, the combination of DIA and FISH had a sensitivity of 70% with a specificity of 82%. In patients with PSC, the sensitivity and specificity of FISH alone and DIA with FISH were 64% and 70%, respectively.[8]

A recent study by Fritcher and colleagues[34] compared the performance of brushings obtained during ERCP in patients with indeterminate strictures using cytology, DIA, and FISH. Of the 498 patients studied, 152 (67%) had CCA and 189 (38%) had PSC. The sensitivity of polysomy FISH (42.9) was significantly higher than cytology (20%) when equivocal cytology was considered negative ($P<.001$) with specificity remaining stable at 99.6%. DIA, on the other hand, was not found to be an independent predictor of malignancy.

Intraductal Ultrasound

Intraductal ultrasound (IDUS) is an endoscopic imaging modality in which high-frequency ultrasound probes are passed at the time of ERCP into the bile duct to obtain detailed images of the bile duct wall and adjacent structures.[36] IDUS has the added advantage of being able to identify local metastases.[36–39] Features suggestive of malignancy include eccentric wall thickening with an irregular surface, hypoechoic mass infiltrating adjacent organs, heterogeneous echo-poor areas invading surrounding tissue, visible lymph nodes, and vascular invasion (**Fig. 3**).[40] Domagk and colleagues[41] compared ERCP with and without IDUS to MRCP. ERCP with IDUS increased the accuracy of malignancy detection from 76% to 88% while the accuracy of MRCP was 58% (P<.05). Stavropoulos and colleagues[42] compared ERCP with and without IDUS and found that the combination increased the accuracy of ERCP from 58% to 90%. Similar results have been shown by others.[43,44] Both formal criteria and the endosonographer's gestalt impression have been compared. For all patients, both interpretations had a sensitivity of about 88% while the specificity was 64% for the formal criteria group and much higher, at 92%, for the gestalt group.[33] In PSC patients, formal criteria were less sensitive and had lower specificity to identify malignant lesions. More importantly, the gestalt group had excellent sensitivity (97%) and specificity (89%) for patients without PSC. The caveat here is that this study was performed at a tertiary care center with a large experience in IDUS, and the results may not be widely applicable.

Per-Oral Cholangioscopy

During ERCP, a small-caliber fiberoptic endoscope can be passed through the working channel of the conventional duodenoscope and allow direct visualization and targeted biopsies of lesions within the bile duct. Features that allow differentiation of benign and malignant biliary strictures have yet to be defined. Fukuda and colleagues[45] studied 97 patients with strictures, of which 38 were malignant. ERCP

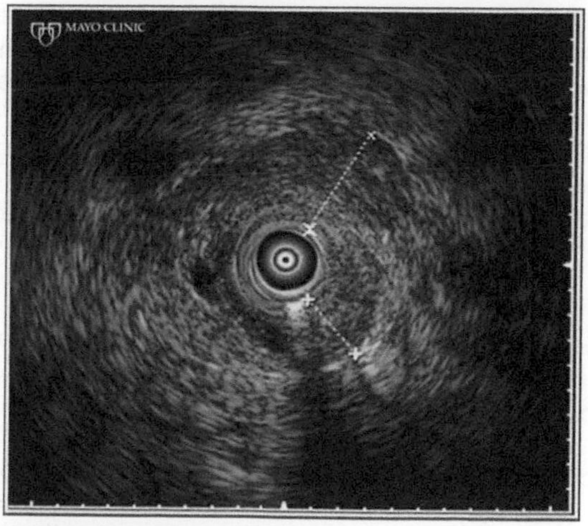

Fig. 3. Intraductal ultrasound image with measurements of the depth of invasion of the cholangiocarcinoma.

with tissue sampling identified 22 of these malignancies, but all were identified with the addition of cholangioscopy without directed biopsies. Thus the sensitivity increased from 57.9% to 100%, but the specificity decreased from 100% to 86.8%. Shah and colleagues[46] performed 72 cholangioscopic procedures on 62 patients. In 53 procedures, cholangioscopy identified an abnormality; in some patients endoscopically directed biopsies were performed while in some cholangiography-assisted biopsies were performed, while both were performed in others. The sensitivity for detection of malignancy was 89% with a specificity of 96%. The 2 missed cancers were intrahepatic CCAs. Tischendorf and colleagues[47] studied 53 patients with PSC and dominant strictures, of whom 12 (23%) had CCA. Cholangioscopic appearance was used to determine malignancy, and cholangiogram-directed biopsies and brushings were obtained. This study showed that cholangioscopy had a higher sensitivity (92% vs 66%) and specificity (93% vs 51%). All 12 malignancies were diagnosed by brushings or biopsies, but 6 patients required more than one ERCP to achieve this. A new single-operator cholangioscope recently became available.[48] In a study of 35 patients, 22 of whom had indeterminate biliary strictures, 20 underwent cholangioscopic-directed biopsies. The sensitivity and specificity for malignancy were 71% and 100%, respectively. However, only 3 patients had CCA.

Hoffman and colleagues[49] studied the use of methylene blue–aided cholangioscopy in 55 patients with biliary strictures, PSC, and post–liver transplant stenoses. The patients first underwent cholangioscopy, followed by methylene blue instillation and repeat cholangioscopy. Some characteristic staining features were seen although further study is warranted. In the authors' institution, narrow band imaging performed during video cholangioscopy is being studied as a method to enhance detection of CCA.

THERAPY

Surgical resection is the only potential for cure for CCA. Surgery with intent to cure has a 5-year survival of 30% to 40% for hilar lesions and 22% to 36% for intrahepatic CCAs.[50] The use of preoperative biliary stenting is controversial. Most patients with distal CCAs do not undergo preoperative stenting. Initial studies showed no benefit from preoperative percutaneous drainage.[51–53] In some studies endoscopic stent placement increases the risk of cholangitis and postoperative infection,[54–57] whereas in others it has decreased morbidity.[58] More recent studies have shown the safety of preoperative biliary drainage.[59–61] Endoscopic nasobiliary drainage allows for effective decompression with a low rate of cholangitis.[62]

Unfortunately, more than half the patients present with unresectable disease, or have advanced liver disease or other comorbidities that preclude surgery.[26] These patients require palliation of biliary obstruction. Endoscopic options include stent placement alone or combined with photodynamic therapy.

Endoscopic Palliation with Stents

In patients with unresectable CCA, jaundice with anorexia and pruritus due to biliary obstruction are the main symptoms that require palliation. Relief of obstruction improves or reduces symptoms and improves quality of life. Ideally, palliative procedures should be minimally invasive, have a low risk of complications, and be cost-effective. Surgical bypass has been compared with endoscopic stent placement.[63–65] Although surgical bypass has longer patency, it is more invasive and less cost-effective for palliation, and is hence reserved for cases where there is complete obstruction of the duct and endoscopic and percutaneous stenting is not possible.

ERCP with biliary stent placement is an effective palliative measure, and is less invasive and painless than percutaneous stenting. However, when access to the bile duct fails or strictures cannot be traversed, the percutaneous approach is the next best option. When deciding the details of the procedure, the location and extent of the biliary obstruction, presence of hepatic lobe atrophy, and life expectancy of the patient must be taken into consideration.[66]

Unilateral versus bilateral stents

In patients with tumors below (distal to) the bifurcation, placement of a single biliary stent is sufficient to relieve jaundice. In hilar CCAs, adequate drainage of a single nonatrophic hepatic lobe is sufficient to achieve resolution of jaundice.[67] The most important concept is that once an obstructed intrahepatic system is contaminated with contrast, it must be drained or there is a high risk of cholangitis. MRCP is useful to evaluate the tumor and hepatic involvement and to determine which lobe to drain during ERCP.[68–70] Minimal contrast is injected until a guide wire has been directed into the ductal system to be drained. A stent is then placed into that system. If multiple metal stents are placed, the distal ends of the stents should approximate each other to allow for future access (**Fig. 4**). Older retrospective studies recommended bilateral stenting for optimal success and improved survival.[71,72] However, in a small prospective study, Hintze and colleagues[70] showed that MRCP-guided ERCP unilateral placement of a single 10-French (10F) biliary stent resulted in resolution of jaundice in 86% of 35 patients. In a landmark article, a prospective study done by De Palma and colleagues[73] in 157 patients (90 with CCA) randomized to unilateral or bilateral stenting, unilateral stenting had a higher rate of technical success (88.6%) and drainage (81%) and lower rate of early complications (18.9%). There was no difference in survival. The same group has also shown similar success with unilaterally placed self-expandable metal stents.[68]

Sizes of stent

Biliary stents become occluded over time. Hence, the smaller the diameter of the stent, the earlier it is likely to occlude. Pedersen[74] retrospectively compared the performance of 7F and 10F stents, and found a trend toward longer patency with the larger diameter stents.

Plastic versus metal stents

Plastic stents have a significantly shorter patency than self-expandable metal stents because of the limited luminal diameter of plastic stents. Once the stent becomes occluded, cholangitis occurs. Hence, plastic stents need to be exchanged every 3 months. Self-expandable metal stents (SEMS) have a much larger internal diameter (up to 30F) and hence remain patent for much longer (**Fig. 5**). Multiple prospective studies[75–80] have compared 10F polyethylene stents to SEMS. SEMS are superior in terms of 30-day outcomes,[81] duration of patency, incidence of cholangitis, number of reinterventions, and hospitalization. Despite SEMS being much more expensive than polyethylene stents, formal cost analyses[66,76,79,82] that account for complications of stent occlusion and need for reinterventions have suggested that SEMS placement is the preferred strategy for patients with a life expectancy of more than 5 to 6 months.

Covered versus uncovered metal stents

Because the commonest cause of stent occlusion in uncovered SEMS is tumor ingrowth, stents were developed with a polyurethane coating. However, it must be noted that covered stents are limited to distal, nonhilar lesions because the covering will occlude branches of the intrahepatic ducts. Prospective studies by Isayama and

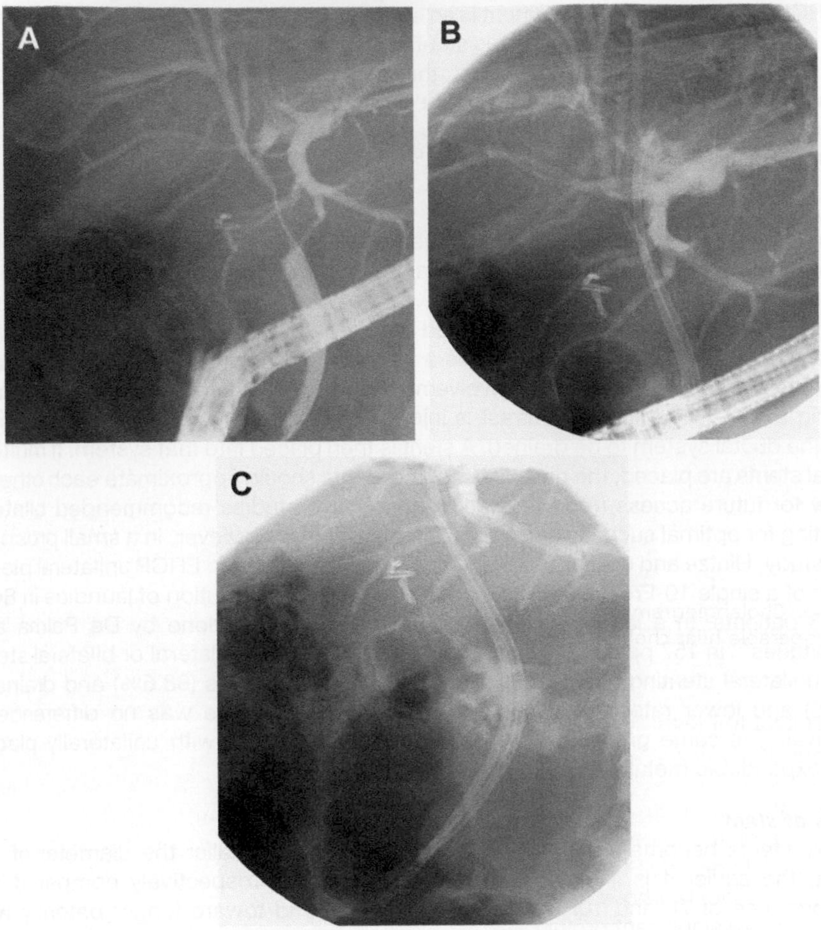

Fig. 4. Cholangiogram of a hilar cholangiocarcinoma before (*A*) and after (*B*) placement of bilateral plastic biliary stents, with distal ends of the stents at the same level (*C*).

colleagues[83] evaluated the efficacy of covered SEMS in palliation of distal malignant biliary strictures. The first study was a pilot nonrandomized study in 21 patients, 3 of whom had CCA. The second study[84] included 112 patients randomized to uncovered or covered stents. Here too, only about 10% of patients had CCA. Based on these limited studies, covered SEMS had superior patency but were associated with an increased incidence of cholecystitis and post-ERCP pancreatitis. Subsequent retrospective cohort series[85,86] comparing the 2 types found no difference in duration of patency. Fumex and colleagues[87] prospectively studied 62 patients (8 CCAs) and found covered SEMS to be effective but with the same patency rate as uncovered stents, but again there was an increased risk of cholecystitis (5 patients) in the covered group. No tumor ingrowth occurred with a median follow-up of 142 days.

Palliation Using Photodynamic Therapy

Photodynamic therapy uses a photosensitizing agent, which is given intravenously and then activated when the neoplastic tissue is illuminated by direct application of

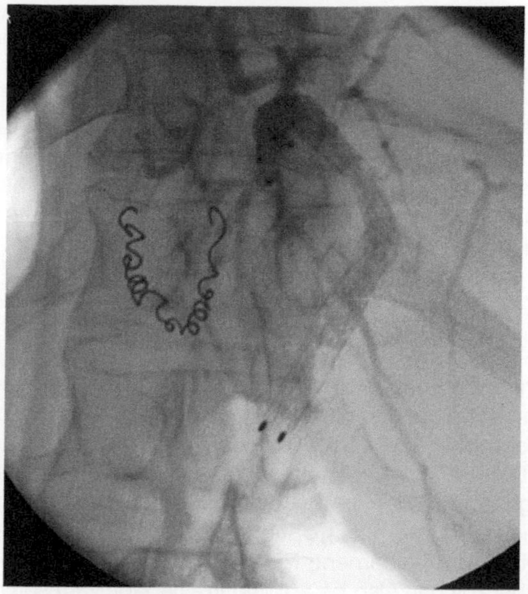

Fig. 5. Cholangiogram showing uncovered metal stent placed in the hilum in a patient with nonoperable hilar cholangiocarcinoma.

laser light to the malignant stricture. Initial nonrandomized studies[88–93] examined the safety, feasibility, and effect of PDT on cholestasis, quality of life, and survival in patients with unresectable CCA. A marked improvement in all these parameters was noted. In these studies, PDT was applied along with placement of plastic biliary stents. Ortner and colleagues[94] prospectively randomized 39 patients with unresectable CCA to receive PDT with plastic stent placement or stent placement alone. A third group of patients who were not randomized also received PDT with stent placement. There was a significant prolongation in survival in patients who received PDT (median 493 days vs 98 days, $P<.0001$). The study was therefore terminated prematurely. Similar results were published by Zoepf and colleagues.[95] The biggest adverse reaction to PDT is skin photosensitivity that usually lasts 6 to 8 weeks. PDT is now routinely used as a palliative therapy in unresectable CCA.

PDT has also been considered for use as an adjuvant[96] and neoadjuvant[97,98] modality, but data for these indications are very limited. The use of PDT with SEMS is being studied in animal models[99] and appears feasible, albeit with adjustments in the light dose.

Intraductal Brachytherapy

Intraductal brachytherapy (IDBT) can be performed endoscopically or percutaneously. Iridium-192 seeds are placed directly across the malignant biliary stricture and the dose of radiation delivered is 10 to 20 Gy. IDBT is usually used along with external beam radiotherapy, and may be employed as a neoadjuvant therapy or as a palliative treatment. There have been varied results with IDBT, with some studies showing an early survival advantage but at a higher complication rate (cholangitis, gastrointestinal bleeding), cost, and hospitalization.[100–102] Other studies[103,104] have shown prolonged survival with low complication rates. Simmons and colleagues[105] studied a novel approach to IDBT in 32 patients undergoing treatment for hilar CCA, and showed that it could safely be performed by passing the catheters via endoscopically placed 10F biliary stents. More prospective randomized studies are required to definitively assess the safety and efficacy of this modality.

High-Intensity Intraductal Ultrasound

Localized ablation of tumor cells can be achieved by using high-intensity intraductal ultrasound delivered during ERCP. Prat and colleagues[106,107] have published the only available data on this modality; in particular, they studied 7 patients with CCA among others and found this method to have promising results in causing tumor cell death. Further studies are needed to confirm this.

SUMMARY

Cholangiocarcinoma is a primary malignancy of the bile ducts, and although rare, the incidence is increasing. The diagnosis is suspected based on radiographic imaging, including cholangiography, but tissue diagnosis is required. Adjunctive diagnostic measures such as DIA, FISH, and per-oral cholangioscopy have been used but require further study. Surgical resection is the only cure, but most patients present at an advanced stage when surgery is not an option. Palliation is then the only option and endoscopic palliation with stent placement, PDT, or brachytherapy is now the standard of care. Endoscopic therapy can also be applied in a neoadjuvant setting in select cases. There is still no consensus on the use of unilateral or bilateral stents, or on the type of stent to be placed. These decisions have to be made on a case by case basis. Endoscopy, however, continues to remain an important component of the therapeutic inventory.

ACKNOWLEDGMENTS

The authors thank Emily Barr-Fritcher, Instructor in Laboratory Medicine/Pathology, Mayo Clinic, Rochester, for DIA and FISH input and images.

REFERENCES

1. Nakeeb A, Pitt HA, Sohn TA, et al. Cholangiocarcinoma. A spectrum of intrahepatic, perihilar, and distal tumors. Ann Surg 1996;224:463.
2. Malhi H, Gores GJ. Cholangiocarcinoma: modern advances in understanding a deadly old disease. J Hepatol 2006;45:856.
3. Lazaridis KN, Gores GJ. Cholangiocarcinoma. Gastroenterology 2005;128:1655.
4. Chapman RW. Risk factors for biliary tract carcinogenesis. Ann Oncol 1999; 10(Suppl 4):308.
5. Sharma MP, Ahuja V. Aetiological spectrum of obstructive jaundice and diagnostic ability of ultrasonography: a clinician's perspective. Trop Gastroenterol 1999;20:167.
6. Manfredi R, Barbaro B, Masselli G, et al. Magnetic resonance imaging of cholangiocarcinoma. Semin Liver Dis 2004;24:155.
7. Manfredi R, Masselli G, Maresca G, et al. MR imaging and MRCP of hilar cholangiocarcinoma. Abdom Imaging 2003;28:319.
8. Gleeson FC, Rajan E, Levy MJ, et al. EUS-guided FNA of regional lymph nodes in patients with unresectable hilar cholangiocarcinoma. Gastrointest Endosc 2008;67:438.
9. Eloubeidi MA, Chen VK, Jhala NC, et al. Endoscopic ultrasound-guided fine needle aspiration biopsy of suspected cholangiocarcinoma. Clin Gastroenterol Hepatol 2004;2:209.

10. Fritscher-Ravens A, Broering DC, Knoefel WT, et al. EUS-guided fine-needle aspiration of suspected hilar cholangiocarcinoma in potentially operable patients with negative brush cytology. Am J Gastroenterol 2004;99:45.
11. Rosch T, Hofrichter K, Frimberger E, et al. ERCP or EUS for tissue diagnosis of biliary strictures? A prospective comparative study. Gastrointest Endosc 2004;60:390.
12. Park MS, Kim TK, Kim KW, et al. Differentiation of extrahepatic bile duct cholangiocarcinoma from benign stricture: findings at MRCP versus ERCP. Radiology 2004;233:234.
13. Glasbrenner B, Ardan M, Boeck W, et al. Prospective evaluation of brush cytology of biliary strictures during endoscopic retrograde cholangiopancreatography. Endoscopy 1999;31:712.
14. Jailwala J, Fogel EL, Sherman S, et al. Triple-tissue sampling at ERCP in malignant biliary obstruction. Gastrointest Endosc 2000;51:383.
15. Macken E, Drijkoningen M, Van Aken E, et al. Brush cytology of ductal strictures during ERCP. Acta Gastroenterol Belg 2000;63:254.
16. Mansfield JC, Griffin SM, Wadehra V, et al. A prospective evaluation of cytology from biliary strictures. Gut 1997;40:671.
17. Pugliese V, Conio M, Nicolo G, et al. Endoscopic retrograde forceps biopsy and brush cytology of biliary strictures: a prospective study. Gastrointest Endosc 1995;42:520.
18. Foutch PG, Kerr DM, Harlan JR, et al. A prospective, controlled analysis of endoscopic cytotechniques for diagnosis of malignant biliary strictures. Am J Gastroenterol 1991;86:577.
19. de Bellis M, Fogel EL, Sherman S, et al. Influence of stricture dilation and repeat brushing on the cancer detection rate of brush cytology in the evaluation of malignant biliary obstruction. Gastrointest Endosc 2003;58:176.
20. Fogel EL, deBellis M, McHenry L, et al. Effectiveness of a new long cytology brush in the evaluation of malignant biliary obstruction: a prospective study. Gastrointest Endosc 2006;63:71.
21. Ponchon T, Gagnon P, Berger F, et al. Value of endobiliary brush cytology and biopsies for the diagnosis of malignant bile duct stenosis: results of a prospective study. Gastrointest Endosc 1995;42:565.
22. Dumonceau JM, Macias Gomez C, Casco C, et al. Grasp or brush for biliary sampling at endoscopic retrograde cholangiography? A blinded randomized controlled trial. Am J Gastroenterol 2008;103:333.
23. Schoefl R, Haefner M, Wrba F, et al. Forceps biopsy and brush cytology during endoscopic retrograde cholangiopancreatography for the diagnosis of biliary stenoses. Scand J Gastroenterol 1997;32:363.
24. Sugiyama M, Atomi Y, Wada N, et al. Endoscopic transpapillary bile duct biopsy without sphincterotomy for diagnosing biliary strictures: a prospective comparative study with bile and brush cytology. Am J Gastroenterol 1996; 91:465.
25. de Bellis M, Sherman S, Fogel EL, et al. Tissue sampling at ERCP in suspected malignant biliary strictures (Part 2). Gastrointest Endosc 2002;56:720.
26. Khan SA, Davidson BR, Goldin R, et al. Guidelines for the diagnosis and treatment of cholangiocarcinoma: consensus document. Gut 2002;51(Suppl 6):VI1.
27. Weber A, von Weyhern C, Fend F, et al. Endoscopic transpapillary brush cytology and forceps biopsy in patients with hilar cholangiocarcinoma. World J Gastroenterol 2008;14:1097.
28. Howell DA, Parsons WG, Jones MA, et al. Complete tissue sampling of biliary strictures at ERCP using a new device. Gastrointest Endosc 1996;43:498.

29. Bergquist A, Tribukait B, Glaumann H, et al. Can DNA cytometry be used for evaluation of malignancy and premalignancy in bile duct strictures in primary sclerosing cholangitis? J Hepatol 2000;33:873.
30. Sebo TJ. Digital image analysis. Mayo Clin Proc 1995;70:81.
31. Baron TH, Harewood GC, Rumalla A, et al. A prospective comparison of digital image analysis and routine cytology for the identification of malignancy in biliary tract strictures. Clin Gastroenterol Hepatol 2004;2:214.
32. Moreno-Luna LE, Kipp B, Halling KC, et al. Advanced cytologic techniques for the detection of malignant pancreatobiliary strictures. Gastroenterology 2006; 131:1064.
33. Levy MJ, Baron TH, Clayton AC, et al. Prospective evaluation of advanced molecular markers and imaging techniques in patients with indeterminate bile duct strictures. Am J Gastroenterol 2008;103:1263.
34. Fritcher EG, Kipp BR, Halling KC, et al: A multivariable model using advanced cytologic methods for the evaluation of indeterminate pancreatobiliary strictures. *Gastroenterology* 136:2180, 2009.
35. Kipp BR, Stadheim LM, Halling SA, et al. A comparison of routine cytology and fluorescence in situ hybridization for the detection of malignant bile duct strictures. Am J Gastroenterol 2004;99:1675.
36. Tamada K, Nagai H, Yasuda Y, et al. Transpapillary intraductal US prior to biliary drainage in the assessment of longitudinal spread of extrahepatic bile duct carcinoma. Gastrointest Endosc 2001;53:300.
37. Tamada K, Ido K, Ueno N, et al. Assessment of hepatic artery invasion by bile duct cancer using intraductal ultrasonography. Endoscopy 1995;27:579.
38. Tamada K, Ido K, Ueno N, et al. Assessment of portal vein invasion by bile duct cancer using intraductal ultrasonography. Endoscopy 1995;27:573.
39. Tamada K, Ido K, Ueno N, et al. Preoperative staging of extrahepatic bile duct cancer with intraductal ultrasonography. Am J Gastroenterol 1995;90:239.
40. Levy MJ, Vazquez-Sequeiros E, Wiersema MJ. Evaluation of the pancreaticobiliary ductal systems by intraductal US. Gastrointest Endosc 2002;55:397.
41. Domagk D, Wessling J, Reimer P, et al. Endoscopic retrograde cholangiopancreatography, intraductal ultrasonography, and magnetic resonance cholangiopancreatography in bile duct strictures: a prospective comparison of imaging diagnostics with histopathological correlation. Am J Gastroenterol 2004;99: 1684.
42. Stavropoulos S, Larghi A, Verna E, et al. Intraductal ultrasound for the evaluation of patients with biliary strictures and no abdominal mass on computed tomography. Endoscopy 2005;37:715.
43. Tamada K, Tomiyama T, Wada S, et al. Endoscopic transpapillary bile duct biopsy with the combination of intraductal ultrasonography in the diagnosis of biliary strictures. Gut 2002;50:326.
44. Vazquez-Sequeiros E, Baron TH, Clain JE, et al. Evaluation of indeterminate bile duct strictures by intraductal US. Gastrointest Endosc 2002;56:372.
45. Fukuda Y, Tsuyuguchi T, Sakai Y, et al. Diagnostic utility of peroral cholangioscopy for various bile-duct lesions. Gastrointest Endosc 2005;62:374.
46. Shah RJ, Langer DA, Antillon MR, et al. Cholangioscopy and cholangioscopic forceps biopsy in patients with indeterminate pancreaticobiliary pathology. Clin Gastroenterol Hepatol 2006;4:219.
47. Tischendorf JJ, Kruger M, Trautwein C, et al. Cholangioscopic characterization of dominant bile duct stenoses in patients with primary sclerosing cholangitis. Endoscopy 2006;38:665.

48. Chen YK, Pleskow DK. SpyGlass single-operator peroral cholangiopancreatoscopy system for the diagnosis and therapy of bile-duct disorders: a clinical feasibility study (with video). Gastrointest Endosc 2007;65:832.
49. Hoffman A, Kiesslich R, Bittinger F, et al. Methylene blue-aided cholangioscopy in patients with biliary strictures: feasibility and outcome analysis. Endoscopy 2008;40:563.
50. Jarnagin WR, Fong Y, DeMatteo RP, et al. Staging, resectability, and outcome in 225 patients with hilar cholangiocarcinoma. Ann Surg 2001;234:507.
51. Hatfield AR, Tobias R, Terblanche J, et al. Preoperative external biliary drainage in obstructive jaundice. A prospective controlled clinical trial. Lancet 1982;2:896.
52. McPherson GA, Benjamin IS, Hodgson HJ, et al. Pre-operative percutaneous transhepatic biliary drainage: the results of a controlled trial. Br J Surg 1984;71:371.
53. Pitt HA, Gomes AS, Lois JF, et al. Does preoperative percutaneous biliary drainage reduce operative risk or increase hospital cost? Ann Surg 1985;201:545.
54. Hochwald SN, Burke EC, Jarnagin WR, et al. Association of preoperative biliary stenting with increased postoperative infectious complications in proximal cholangiocarcinoma. Arch Surg 1999;134:261.
55. Jagannath P, Dhir V, Shrikhande S, et al. Effect of preoperative biliary stenting on immediate outcome after pancreaticoduodenectomy. Br J Surg 2005;92:356.
56. Pisters PW, Hudec WA, Hess KR, et al. Effect of preoperative biliary decompression on pancreaticoduodenectomy-associated morbidity in 300 consecutive patients. Ann Surg 2001;234:47.
57. Sohn TA, Yeo CJ, Cameron JL, et al. Do preoperative biliary stents increase postpancreaticoduodenectomy complications? J Gastrointest Surg 2000;4:258.
58. Cherqui D, Benoist S, Malassagne B, et al. Major liver resection for carcinoma in jaundiced patients without preoperative biliary drainage. Arch Surg 2000;135:302.
59. Hemming AW, Reed AI, Fujita S, et al. Surgical management of hilar cholangiocarcinoma. Ann Surg 2005;241:693.
60. Kawasaki S, Imamura H, Kobayashi A, et al. Results of surgical resection for patients with hilar bile duct cancer: application of extended hepatectomy after biliary drainage and hemihepatic portal vein embolization. Ann Surg 2003;238:84.
61. Sano T, Shimada K, Sakamoto Y, et al. One hundred two consecutive hepatobiliary resections for perihilar cholangiocarcinoma with zero mortality. Ann Surg 2006;244:240.
62. Arakura N, Takayama M, Ozaki Y, et al. Efficacy of preoperative endoscopic nasobiliary drainage for hilar cholangiocarcinoma. J Hepatobiliary Pancreat Surg 2009;16:473–7.
63. Martin RC 2nd, Vitale GC, Reed DN, et al. Cost comparison of endoscopic stenting vs surgical treatment for unresectable cholangiocarcinoma. Surg Endosc 2002;16:667.
64. Smith AC, Dowsett JF, Russell RC, et al. Randomised trial of endoscopic stenting versus surgical bypass in malignant low bile duct obstruction. Lancet 1994;344:1655.
65. Sunpaweravong S, Ovartlarnporn B, Khow-ean U, et al. Endoscopic stenting versus surgical bypass in advanced malignant distal bile duct obstruction: cost-effectiveness analysis. Asian J Surg 2005;28:262.

66. Levy MJ, Baron TH, Gostout CJ, et al. Palliation of malignant extrahepatic biliary obstruction with plastic versus expandable metal stents: an evidence-based approach. Clin Gastroenterol Hepatol 2004;2:273.
67. Baer HU, Rhyner M, Stain SC, et al. The effect of communication between the right and left liver on the outcome of surgical drainage for jaundice due to malignant obstruction at the hilus of the liver. HPB Surg 1994;8:27.
68. De Palma GD, Pezzullo A, Rega M, et al. Unilateral placement of metallic stents for malignant hilar obstruction: a prospective study. Gastrointest Endosc 2003;58:50.
69. Freeman ML, Overby C. Selective MRCP and CT-targeted drainage of malignant hilar biliary obstruction with self-expanding metallic stents. Gastrointest Endosc 2003;58:41.
70. Hintze RE, Abou-Rebyeh H, Adler A, et al. Magnetic resonance cholangiopancreatography-guided unilateral endoscopic stent placement for Klatskin tumors. Gastrointest Endosc 2001;53:40.
71. Chang WH, Kortan P, Haber GB. Outcome in patients with bifurcation tumors who undergo unilateral versus bilateral hepatic duct drainage. Gastrointest Endosc 1998;47:354.
72. Deviere J, Baize M, de Toeuf J, et al. Long-term follow-up of patients with hilar malignant stricture treated by endoscopic internal biliary drainage. Gastrointest Endosc 1988;34:95.
73. De Palma GD, Galloro G, Siciliano S, et al. Unilateral versus bilateral endoscopic hepatic duct drainage in patients with malignant hilar biliary obstruction: results of a prospective, randomized, and controlled study. Gastrointest Endosc 2001;53:547.
74. Pedersen FM. Endoscopic management of malignant biliary obstruction. Is stent size of 10 French gauge better than 7 French gauge? Scand J Gastroenterol 1993;28:185.
75. Davids PH, Groen AK, Rauws EA, et al. Randomised trial of self-expanding metal stents versus polyethylene stents for distal malignant biliary obstruction. Lancet 1992;340:1488.
76. Kaassis M, Boyer J, Dumas R, et al. Plastic or metal stents for malignant stricture of the common bile duct? Results of a randomized prospective study. Gastrointest Endosc 2003;57:178.
77. Knyrim K, Wagner HJ, Pausch J, et al. A prospective, randomized, controlled trial of metal stents for malignant obstruction of the common bile duct. Endoscopy 1993;25:207.
78. Prat F, Chapat O, Ducot B, et al. A randomized trial of endoscopic drainage methods for inoperable malignant strictures of the common bile duct. Gastrointest Endosc 1998;47:1.
79. Soderlund C, Linder S. Covered metal versus plastic stents for malignant common bile duct stenosis: a prospective, randomized, controlled trial. Gastrointest Endosc 2006;63:986.
80. Wagner HJ, Knyrim K, Vakil N, et al. Plastic endoprostheses versus metal stents in the palliative treatment of malignant hilar biliary obstruction. A prospective and randomized trial. Endoscopy 1993;25:213.
81. Perdue DG, Freeman ML, DiSario JA, et al. Plastic versus self-expanding metallic stents for malignant hilar biliary obstruction: a prospective multicenter observational cohort study. J Clin Gastroenterol 2008;42:1040.
82. Yeoh KG, Zimmerman MJ, Cunningham JT, et al. Comparative costs of metal versus plastic biliary stent strategies for malignant obstructive jaundice by decision analysis. Gastrointest Endosc 1999;49:466.

83. Isayama H, Komatsu Y, Tsujino T, et al. Polyurethane-covered metal stent for management of distal malignant biliary obstruction. Gastrointest Endosc 2002; 55:366.
84. Isayama H, Komatsu Y, Tsujino T, et al. A prospective randomised study of "covered" versus "uncovered" diamond stents for the management of distal malignant biliary obstruction. Gut 2004;53:729.
85. Park do H, Kim MH, Choi JS, et al. Covered versus uncovered wallstent for malignant extrahepatic biliary obstruction: a cohort comparative analysis. Clin Gastroenterol Hepatol 2006;4:790.
86. Yoon WJ, Lee JK, Lee KH, et al. A comparison of covered and uncovered Wallstents for the management of distal malignant biliary obstruction. Gastrointest Endosc 2006;63:996.
87. Fumex F, Coumaros D, Napoleon B, et al. Similar performance but higher cholecystitis rate with covered biliary stents: results from a prospective multicenter evaluation. Endoscopy 2006;38:787.
88. Berr F, Wiedmann M, Tannapfel A, et al. Photodynamic therapy for advanced bile duct cancer: evidence for improved palliation and extended survival. Hepatology 2000;31:291.
89. Dumoulin FL, Gerhardt T, Fuchs S, et al. Phase II study of photodynamic therapy and metal stent as palliative treatment for nonresectable hilar cholangiocarcinoma. Gastrointest Endosc 2003;57:860.
90. Harewood GC, Baron TH, Rumalla A, et al. Pilot study to assess patient outcomes following endoscopic application of photodynamic therapy for advanced cholangiocarcinoma. J Gastroenterol Hepatol 2005;20:415.
91. McCaughan JS Jr, Mertens BF, Cho C, et al. Photodynamic therapy to treat tumors of the extrahepatic biliary ducts. A case report. Arch Surg 1991;126:111.
92. Ortner MA, Liebetruth J, Schreiber S, et al. Photodynamic therapy of nonresectable cholangiocarcinoma. Gastroenterology 1998;114:536.
93. Rumalla A, Baron TH, Wang KK, et al. Endoscopic application of photodynamic therapy for cholangiocarcinoma. Gastrointest Endosc 2001;53:500.
94. Ortner ME, Caca K, Berr F, et al. Successful photodynamic therapy for nonresectable cholangiocarcinoma: a randomized prospective study. Gastroenterology 2003;125:1355.
95. Zoepf T, Jakobs R, Arnold JC, et al. Palliation of nonresectable bile duct cancer: improved survival after photodynamic therapy. Am J Gastroenterol 2005;100: 2426.
96. Nanashima A, Yamaguchi H, Shibasaki S, et al. Adjuvant photodynamic therapy for bile duct carcinoma after surgery: a preliminary study. J Gastroenterol 2004; 39:1095.
97. Berr F, Tannapfel A, Lamesch P, et al. Neoadjuvant photodynamic therapy before curative resection of proximal bile duct carcinoma. J Hepatol 2000;32: 352.
98. Wiedmann M, Caca K, Berr F, et al. Neoadjuvant photodynamic therapy as a new approach to treating hilar cholangiocarcinoma: a phase II pilot study. Cancer 2003;97:2783.
99. Wang LW, Li LB, Li ZS, et al. Self-expandable metal stents and trans-stent light delivery: are metal stents and photodynamic therapy compatible? Lasers Surg Med 2008;40:651.
100. Bowling TE, Galbraith SM, Hatfield AR, et al. A retrospective comparison of endoscopic stenting alone with stenting and radiotherapy in non-resectable cholangiocarcinoma. Gut 1996;39:852.

101. Foo ML, Gunderson LL, Bender CE, et al. External radiation therapy and transcatheter iridium in the treatment of extrahepatic bile duct carcinoma. Int J Radiat Oncol Biol Phys 1997;39:929.
102. Gerhards MF, van Gulik TM, Gonzalez Gonzalez D, et al. Results of postoperative radiotherapy for resectable hilar cholangiocarcinoma. World J Surg 2003; 27:173.
103. Valek V, Kysela P, Kala Z, et al. Brachytherapy and percutaneous stenting in the treatment of cholangiocarcinoma: a prospective randomised study. Eur J Radiol 2007;62:175.
104. Bruha R, Petrtyl J, Kubecova M, et al. Intraluminal brachytherapy and selfexpandable stents in nonresectable biliary malignancies—the question of long-term palliation. Hepatogastroenterology 2001;48:631.
105. Simmons DT, Baron TH, Petersen BT, et al. A novel endoscopic approach to brachytherapy in the management of Hilar cholangiocarcinoma. Am J Gastroenterol 2006;101:1792.
106. Prat F, Lafon C, De Lima DM, et al. Endoscopic treatment of cholangiocarcinoma and carcinoma of the duodenal papilla by intraductal high-intensity US: results of a pilot study. Gastrointest Endosc 2002;56:909.
107. Prat F, Lafon C, Theilliere JY, et al. Destruction of a bile duct carcinoma by intraductal high intensity ultrasound during ERCP. Gastrointest Endosc 2001;53:797.

Endoscopic Retrograde Cholangiopancreatography in Diagnosis and Treatment of Primary Sclerosing Cholangitis

Daniel Gotthardt, MD*, Adolf Stiehl, MD

KEYWORDS

- Sclerosing cholangitis
- Endoscopic retrograde cholangiopancreatography
- Endoscopic therapy • Dominant stenosis
- Cholangiocarcinoma

Progressive fibrosing inflammation leading to multiple stenoses of intra- and/or extrahepatic bile ducts is characteristic of primary sclerosing cholangitis (PSC)[1–4]; this leads to cholestasis and finally to cirrhosis of the liver. In early stages only alkaline phosphatase (AP) and γ-glutamyl transferase (GGT) are elevated, whereas increased bilirubin is found only in advanced disease. Stenoses of major bile ducts lead to biliary obstruction with all consequences of severe cholestatic disease. Besides jaundice and pruritus, important complications are biliary infection, stone formation proximal of the stenosis, and parenchymal liver damage.

DIAGNOSIS OF DOMINANT STENOSES: ERCP OR MRCP?

A total or subtotal stenosis of the common duct (<1.5 mm) or of the left or right hepatic duct (<1.0 mm) close to the bifurcation may lead to cholestasis with consecutive damage of the drained liver tissue. Such stenoses are termed dominant stenoses.

PSC is routinely diagnosed by endoscopic retrograde cholangiography (ERC) or alternatively by magnetic resonance cholangiography (MRC), both of which show multiple stenoses of intra- and/or extrahepatic bile ducts. In experienced centers magnetic resonance cholangiopancreatography (MRCP) allows the detection of

Department of Medicine IV, University of Heidelberg, Im Neuenheimer Feld 410, Heidelberg 69120, Germany
* Corresponding author.
E-mail address: daniel_gotthardt@med.uni-heidelberg.de

Clin Liver Dis 14 (2010) 349–358
doi:10.1016/j.cld.2010.03.010

PSC with a sensitivity of 83% to 88% and specificity of 92% to 99% (**Table 1**), and these figures are considered excellent,[5–7] Although there are no specific data available on the sensitivity and specificity of MRC in detecting dominant stenoses requiring endoscopic opening, the figures for the detection of dominant stenoses are expected to be similar to those for the detection of PSC. Because the diagnosis of PSC, and the detection of patients with dominant stenoses in particular, require the lifelong surveillance and treatment of the patient, a definite diagnosis is needed. A sensitivity and specificity of a diagnostic technique yielding about 90% appear good, but still do not seem satisfactory because this means that 1 out of 10 diagnoses are false positive or false negative, with possible dramatic consequences for the individual patient. It seems likely that with further improvement of imaging methods and especially the introduction of 3-dimensional magnetic resonance cholangiopancreatography (MRCP), the situation will further advance. Using this technique a recent study achieved a specificity of 88% and a sensitivity of 99%,[7] though another more recent study reported slightly less specificity and sensitivity of 77% and 86%, respectively.[8] Although these figures appear promising, in many cases at present an ERCP is still required for the correct decision in the treatment strategy. Thus up to now, despite progress and excellent expertise in MRCP technique in many centers, ERCP remains the gold standard.

PREVALENCE AND INCIDENCE OF DOMINANT STENOSES

During long-term follow-up of patients with PSC, dominant stenoses develop frequently (**Table 2**). In a prospective trial on the effect of ursodeoxycholic acid (UDCA) on bile duct disease in patients with PSC, in whom repeat cholangiographies were performed during treatment with UDCA for 8 years, 35% of the patients had or developed at least one dominant stenosis of major bile ducts.[9] In the consecutive study, over 13 years 50% of the patients had developed dominant stenoses.[10] This ratio has been confirmed in other studies, ranging from 35.6% to 56.9%,[11–13] underlining that depending on disease activity, more and more patients have dominant stenoses.

This situation holds especially true for patients showing fibrosing inflammation in liver histology (stages 2–4), who increasingly showed obstruction of major bile ducts.[10] On the other hand, patients without fibrosis in liver histology (stage 1) developed dominant stenoses infrequently while under UDCA treatment. Thus it appears possible that UDCA decreases or slows down this process but could not prevent it. Patients with dominant stenoses of major bile ducts need to be referred for endoscopic treatment, which may be highly effective (**Table 3**).[10,14–22]

Table 1
Sensitivity and specificity of magnetic resonance cholangiography in primary sclerosing cholangitis

Study	Patients (n)	Sensitivity (%)	Specificity (%)
Fulcher et al, 2000[5]	34	85–88	92–97
Angulo et al, 2000[6]	23	83	98
Textor et al, 2002[7]	34	88	99
Berstad et al, 2006[51]	39	80	87
Weber et al, 2008[8]	69	86	77

Table 2
Prevalence of dominant stenoses in patients with primary sclerosing cholangitis

Study	Patients (n)	Dominant Stenoses (n)	Dominant Stenoses (%)
Stiehl et al, 2002[10]	106	53	50.0
Bjornsson et al, 2004[12]	125	56	44.8
Tischendorf et al, 2007[11]	273	98	35.9
Gluck et al, 2008[13]	117	59	50.4
Rudolph et al, 2009[32]	171	97	56.7

ENDOSCOPIC VERSUS SURGICAL VERSUS PERCUTANEOUS TREATMENT OF DOMINANT STENOSES

Historically, dominant stenoses had been treated surgically. The first nonsurgical attempts to treat biliary strictures interventionally were made via the percutaneous route. Stenoses commonly were dilated and afterwards percutaneous drains were placed for up to 3 months. Many patients benefited from these procedures but developed recurrent symptoms after 6 to 18 months.[23] Because repeated interventions are regularly needed (see **Table 3**) the endoscopic management evolved to become the preferred method over the surgical as well as the percutaneous radiological approaches. The advantages of endoscopy were the possibility of repeated interventions with a low complication rate.[24]

Endoscopic treatment allows rapid opening of dominant stenoses. After endoscopic dilatation of dominant stenoses aspartate aminotransferase, AP, GGT, and serum bilirubin decrease. In the majority of patients, this improvement of laboratory parameters of cholestasis is accompanied by a decrease of jaundice and also of pruritus if present.

Table 3
Endoscopic treatment of strictures in patients with primary sclerosing cholangitis

Study	Patients (n)	Stents Placed (n)	Dilatations Performed (n)	Biochemical Response	Improved Survival[a]
Johnson et al, 1987[15]	35	11	24	+	N/A
Gaing et al, 1993[17]	16	15	6	N/A	N/A
Lee et al, 1995[18]	53	38	50	+	N/A
van Milligen de Wit et al, 1996[19]	25	21	0	+	N/A
Wagner et al, 1996[20]	12	0	12	+	N/A
Kaya et al, 2001[21]	71	37	34	+	N/A
Baluyut et al, 2001[22]	63	32	140	+	+
Stiehl et al, 2002[10]	52	5	210	+	+
Gluck et al, 2008[13]	84	84	160	+	+

Abbreviations: N/A not analyzed in this study; +/–/0, positive/negative/no influence of endoscopic treatment on biochemical parameters or survival.
[a] Compared with predicted survival by Mayo Risk Score.

Because the percutaneous approach is associated with a higher complication rate, it is therefore only indicated if the endoscopic access is not possible. In experienced centers endoscopic interventions represent the treatment of choice and operative measures, that is, choledochojejunostomy no longer plays a role. In fact it has been shown that surgical treatment of the biliary tract in these patients might worsen outcome after liver transplantation.[25]

WHY TREAT PATIENTS WITH DOMINANT STENOSES ENDOSCOPICALLY?

Biliary strictures of any etiology inhibit bile flow, increase biliary back pressure, and therefore may lead to progressive deterioration of liver function and terminally to cirrhosis. In addition, patients with biliary strictures are prone to have bacterial cholangitis.[26,27] This infection itself in addition probably contributes to the liver damage. In analogy to patients with biliary obstruction due to pancreatitis, biliary decompression may stop progression of liver disease and may even lead to regression of fibrosis.[28] Based on these findings, patients with significant biliary obstruction should be treated as early as possible, because it seems highly probable that relief of biliary obstruction by opening of dominant stenoses in PSC has beneficial effects on liver function and morphology.

BALLOON DILATATION AND STENTING OF DOMINANT STENOSES

If strictures of the larger bile ducts are detected by ERC, early endoscopic intervention is obligatory. Either balloon dilatation or stenting may be used to treat bile duct stenosis (see **Table 3**). As the first step the authors recommend only a small endoscopic papillotomy. Because a complete sphincterotomy eases ascending infection of the bile ducts, it hence appears crucial that a small and not a wide papillotomy is performed. Then high-grade stenoses can be passed by a Terumo guide wire. The Terumo guide wire has the advantage of a very flexible tip that helps to prevent perforation of an inflamed bile duct. Afterwards stiff dilatation from 5F up to 7F allows the introduction of a balloon dilator for the dilatation up to 18F or 24F. The ideal goal is to dilate the common duct to 18F or, even better, 24F, and to dilate the hepatic ducts up to 18F.[10] Because continuing inflammation leads to reocclusion of the bile ducts in most cases, repeated endoscopic intervention is necessary to keep the stenosis open. This phenomenon most likely results from the fact that the fiber ring around the bile duct responsible for the stenosis has the tendency to shrink, resulting in the reocclusion. In a few patients it is not possible to open a total stenosis primarily by the endoscopic route. In these patients a combined percutaneous and endoscopic approach may be tried to achieve the dilatation of the bile ducts. Due to the high risk of bacterial infection, these endoscopic procedures should be performed under antibiotic prophylaxis.[26]

The first attempts to treat dominant stenoses in PSC endoscopically were made by placement of stents into the stenosis that were kept there for variable periods of time.[14] After endoscopic papillotomy and graded dilatation as described before, a guide wire is placed and stents of up to 11F are introduced over this wire. A frequent problem of this procedure is the early occlusion of these plastic stents by inflammatory material, mainly cell debris, which is shed from the bile ducts. In PSC, as in patients after liver transplantation,[29] these stents occlude early. Because this occlusion of the stent leads to bacterial infection of the proximal biliary tree, stents in general should be removed or replaced within a short period of time.[30]

The advantage of stenting is prevention of rapid reocclusion of the impaired bile duct. A disadvantage of stenting, on the other hand, lies in the fact that actually 2 endoscopic interventions have to be performed, one to introduce and then one to remove the stent. The net effect is the dilatation of the stenosis up to 11F. Due to the continuous shedding of cells and secretion in chronic inflammation in many PSC patients, the stents occlude early and replacement has to be performed within weeks. Stent occlusion is a severe problem because it predisposes to biliary infection, which represents a serious issue in patients with dominant stenoses.[27] In addition, an occluded stent allows even less bile flow than the native bile duct, thereby leading to biliary obstruction and aggravating cholestasis. Moreover, in patients with dominant stenoses close to the bifurcation, the stenting of one hepatic duct often hinders the bile flow inside the other hepatic duct, and in patients with a rudimental hepatic duct it will not be possible to stent both hepatic ducts. These considerations were verified in a study evaluating the effect of stenting. After balloon dilatation of dominant stenoses additional stenting was no more effective and was associated with more complications.[21] Therefore in the more recent studies, balloon dilatation has become the method of choice for endoscopic therapy.[10,20,22]

BEYOND AND WITHIN THE MEANS OF ENDOSCOPIC TREATMENT

Initially, only stenoses of the common duct were treated endoscopically and this was applied to short strictures only. There is increasing evidence that long-segment stenoses of the common bile duct of over 2 cm length also may be treated, with excellent results.[10] In fact in this study, the majority of patients dilated for dominant stenoses had long segment stenoses. In most cases one single dilatation is not sufficient, and repeated dilatations over years are necessary until the duct remains open.

After successful reopening of the common bile duct, many patients in addition accrue dominant stenoses of the hepatic ducts. The treatment of these stenoses then exhibits an important challenge. Again, attempts to treat such stenoses by endoscopic means showed that shorter-segment stenoses within 2 cm of the bifurcation may be treated by dilatation, with very good results.[10] In the aforementioned study the vast majority of cases (87.5%) were able to be treated and it was possible to open at least one (the right or the left) dominant short-segment stenosis of a hepatic duct. Most attempts to open long-segment stenoses of the hepatic ducts were not successful. Therefore, only short-segment stenoses of the hepatic ducts located within 2 cm of the bifurcation are considered to be treated effectively. For all other high-grade stenoses located more proximal of the biliary tree, endoscopic treatment options are very limited. High-grade intrahepatic stenoses situated more than 2 cm above the bifurcation develop with progression of disease more frequently. The appearance of such stenoses indicates advancement of PSC, in turn indicating the upcoming requirement of liver transplantation.

Dilatation performed by an experienced endoscopist appears a far more effective form of endoscopic treatment than stenting. In patients with biliary sepsis, however, temporary stenting for a very short period of time may be indicated, because rapid reocclusion of the duct is likely to happen more frequently in this setting and, in addition, has a high risk of morbidity and mortality in this subgroup of patients. During long-term follow up, dilatation of the common duct was very successful. As shown recently 5 and 10 years after the first dilatation of a dominant stenosis, 81 and 52% of the patients were alive free of liver transplantation.[31] Clinical progression of the disease that ultimately led to liver transplantation usually was associated with progressive obstruction of multiple intrahepatic bile ducts, in which endoscopic treatment is of limited success, whereas stenoses of the extrahepatic ducts generally should be opened, thereby relieving cholestasis.

- Endoscopic treatment has been shown to improve biochemical parameters and actuarial survival compared with predicted survival.
- Treatment of choice is balloon dilatation. Stent placement may be indicated if rapid reocclusion of the bile duct with sepsis is imminent.
- Every endoscopic intervention should be performed under antibiotic prophylaxis.
- Endoscopic brushing and biopsy as well as bile analysis are important for detection of cholangiocarcinoma.

All recommendations are Grade B.

REFERENCES

1. Chapman RW, Arborgh BA, Rhodes JM, et al. Primary sclerosing cholangitis: a review of its clinical features, cholangiography, and hepatic histology. Gut 1980;21:870.
2. Wiesner RH, Grambsch PM, Dickson ER, et al. Primary sclerosing cholangitis: natural history, prognostic factors and survival analysis. Hepatology 1989;10:430.
3. Farrant JM, Hayllar KM, Wilkinson ML, et al. Natural history and prognostic variables in primary sclerosing cholangitis. Gastroenterology 1991;100:1710.
4. Broome U, Olsson R, Loof L, et al. Natural history and prognostic factors in 305 Swedish patients with primary sclerosing cholangitis. Gut 1996;38:610.
5. Fulcher AS, Turner MA, Franklin KJ, et al. Primary sclerosing cholangitis: evaluation with MR cholangiography—a case-control study. Radiology 2000;215:71.
6. Angulo P, Pearce DH, Johnson CD, et al. Magnetic resonance cholangiography in patients with biliary disease: its role in primary sclerosing cholangitis. J Hepatol 2000;33:520.
7. Textor HJ, Flacke S, Pauleit D, et al. Three-dimensional magnetic resonance cholangiopancreatography with respiratory triggering in the diagnosis of primary sclerosing cholangitis: comparison with endoscopic retrograde cholangiography. Endoscopy 2002;34:984.
8. Weber C, Kuhlencordt R, Grotelueschen R, et al. Magnetic resonance cholangiopancreatography in the diagnosis of primary sclerosing cholangitis. Endoscopy 2008;40:739.
9. Stiehl A, Rudolph G, Sauer P, et al. Efficacy of ursodeoxycholic acid treatment and endoscopic dilation of major duct stenoses in primary sclerosing cholangitis. An 8-year prospective study. J Hepatol 1997;26:560.
10. Stiehl A, Rudolph G, Kloters-Plachky P, et al. Development of dominant bile duct stenoses in patients with primary sclerosing cholangitis treated with ursodeoxycholic acid: outcome after endoscopic treatment. J Hepatol 2002;36:151.
11. Tischendorf JJ, Hecker H, Kruger M, et al. Characterization, outcome, and prognosis in 273 patients with primary sclerosing cholangitis: a single center study. Am J Gastroenterol 2007;102:107.
12. Bjornsson E, Lindqvist-Ottosson J, Asztely M, et al. Dominant strictures in patients with primary sclerosing cholangitis. Am J Gastroenterol 2004;99:502.
13. Gluck M, Cantone NR, Brandabur JJ, et al. A twenty-year experience with endoscopic therapy for symptomatic primary sclerosing cholangitis. J Clin Gastroenterol 2008;42:1032.
14. Grijm R, Huibregtse K, Bartelsman J, et al. Therapeutic investigations in primary sclerosing cholangitis. Dig Dis Sci 1986;31:792.

15. Johnson GK, Geenen JE, Venu RP, et al. Endoscopic treatment of biliary duct strictures in sclerosing cholangitis: follow-up assessment of a new therapeutic approach. Gastrointest Endosc 1987;33:9.
16. Cotton PB, Nickl N. Endoscopic and radiologic approaches to therapy in primary sclerosing cholangitis. Semin Liver Dis 1991;11:40.
17. Gaing AA, Geders JM, Cohen SA, et al. Endoscopic management of primary sclerosing cholangitis: review, and report of an open series. Am J Gastroenterol 1993;88:2000.
18. Lee JG, Schutz SM, England RE, et al. Endoscopic therapy of sclerosing cholangitis. Hepatology 1995;21:661.
19. van Milligen de Wit AW, van Bracht J, Rauws EA, et al. Endoscopic stent therapy for dominant extrahepatic bile duct strictures in primary sclerosing cholangitis. Gastrointest Endosc 1996;44:293.
20. Wagner S, Gebel M, Meier P, et al. Endoscopic management of biliary tract strictures in primary sclerosing cholangitis. Endoscopy 1996;28:546.
21. Kaya M, Petersen BT, Angulo P, et al. Balloon dilation compared to stenting of dominant strictures in primary sclerosing cholangitis. Am J Gastroenterol 2001; 96:1059.
22. Baluyut AR, Sherman S, Lehman GA, et al. Impact of endoscopic therapy on the survival of patients with primary sclerosing cholangitis. Gastrointest Endosc 2001;53:308.
23. May GR, Bender CE, LaRusso NF, et al. Nonoperative dilatation of dominant strictures in primary sclerosing cholangitis. AJR Am J Roentgenol 1985;145:1061.
24. Bangarulingam SY, Gossard AA, Petersen BT, et al. Complications of endoscopic retrograde cholangiopancreatography in primary sclerosing cholangitis. Am J Gastroenterol 2009;104:855–60.
25. Farges O, Malassagne B, Sebagh M, et al. Primary sclerosing cholangitis: liver transplantation or biliary surgery. Surgery 1995;117:146.
26. Olsson R, Bjornsson E, Backman L, et al. Bile duct bacterial isolates in primary sclerosing cholangitis: a study of explanted livers. J Hepatol 1998;28:426.
27. Pohl J, Ring A, Stremmel W, et al. The role of dominant stenoses in bacterial infections of bile ducts in primary sclerosing cholangitis. Eur J Gastroenterol Hepatol 2006;18:69.
28. Hammel P, Couvelard A, O'Toole D, et al. Regression of liver fibrosis after biliary drainage in patients with chronic pancreatitis and stenosis of the common bile duct. N Engl J Med 2001;344:418.
29. Kulaksiz H, Weiss KH, Gotthardt D, et al. Is stenting necessary after balloon dilation of post-transplantation biliary strictures? Results of a prospective comparative study. Endoscopy 2008;40:746.
30. Ponsioen CY, Lam K, van Milligen de Wit AW, et al. Four years experience with short term stenting in primary sclerosing cholangitis. Am J Gastroenterol 1999; 94:2403.
31. Gotthardt DN, Rudolph G, Klöters-Plachky P, et al. Endoscopic dilation of dominant stenoses in primary sclerosing cholangitis: outcome after long-term treatment. Gastrointest Endosc 2010;71:527–34.
32. Rudolph G, Gotthardt D, Kloters-Plachky P, et al. Influence of dominant bile duct stenoses and biliary infections on outcome in primary sclerosing cholangitis. J Hepatol 2009;51:149–55.
33. Farkkila M, Karvonen AL, Nurmi H, et al. Metronidazole and ursodeoxycholic acid for primary sclerosing cholangitis: a randomized placebo-controlled trial. Hepatology 2004;40:1379.

34. Hultcrantz R, Olsson R, Danielsson A, et al. A 3-year prospective study on serum tumor markers used for detecting cholangiocarcinoma in patients with primary sclerosing cholangitis. J Hepatol 1999;30:669.
35. Keiding S, Hansen SB, Rasmussen HH, et al. Detection of cholangiocarcinoma in primary sclerosing cholangitis by positron emission tomography. Hepatology 1998;28:700.
36. Kluge R, Schmidt F, Caca K, et al. Positron emission tomography with [(18)F]fluoro-2-deoxy-D-glucose for diagnosis and staging of bile duct cancer. Hepatology 2001;33:1029.
37. Ponsioen CY, Vrouenraets SM, van Milligen de Wit AW, et al. Value of brush cytology for dominant strictures in primary sclerosing cholangitis. Endoscopy 1999;31:305.
38. Boberg KM, Jebsen P, Clausen OP, et al. Diagnostic benefit of biliary brush cytology in cholangiocarcinoma in primary sclerosing cholangitis. J Hepatol 2006;45:568.
39. Charatcharoenwitthaya P, Enders FB, Halling KC, et al. Utility of serum tumor markers, imaging, and biliary cytology for detecting cholangiocarcinoma in primary sclerosing cholangitis. Hepatology 2008;48:1106.
40. Rudolph G, Kloeters-Plachky P, Rost D, et al. The incidence of cholangiocarcinoma in primary sclerosing cholangitis after long-time treatment with ursodeoxycholic acid. Eur J Gastroenterol Hepatol 2007;19:487.
41. Burak K, Angulo P, Pasha TM, et al. Incidence and risk factors for cholangiocarcinoma in primary sclerosing cholangitis. Am J Gastroenterol 2004;99:523.
42. Beuers U, Spengler U, Kruis W, et al. Ursodeoxycholic acid for treatment of primary sclerosing cholangitis: a placebo-controlled trial. Hepatology 1992;16:707.
43. Stiehl A, Walker S, Stiehl L, et al. Effect of ursodeoxycholic acid on liver and bile duct disease in primary sclerosing cholangitis. A 3-year pilot study with a placebo-controlled study period. J Hepatol 1994;20:57.
44. Mitchell SA, Bansi DS, Hunt N, et al. A preliminary trial of high-dose ursodeoxycholic acid in primary sclerosing cholangitis. Gastroenterology 2001;121:900.
45. Lindor KD. Ursodiol for primary sclerosing cholangitis. Mayo Primary Sclerosing Cholangitis-Ursodeoxycholic Acid Study Group. N Engl J Med 1997;336:691.
46. Harnois DM, Angulo P, Jorgensen RA, et al. High-dose ursodeoxycholic acid as a therapy for patients with primary sclerosing cholangitis. Am J Gastroenterol 2001;96:1558.
47. Cullen SN, Rust C, Fleming K, et al. High dose ursodeoxycholic acid for the treatment of primary sclerosing cholangitis is safe and effective. J Hepatol 2008;48:792.
48. Lindor KD, Enders FB, Schmoll JA, et al. Randomized, double-blind controlled trial of high-dose ursodeoxycholic acid (UDCA) for primary sclerosing cholangitis (PSC). Hepatology 2008;48:LB2.
49. Silveira MG, Torok NJ, Gossard AA, et al. Minocycline in the treatment of patients with primary sclerosing cholangitis: results of a pilot study. Am J Gastroenterol 2009;104:83.
50. Alabraba E, Nightingale P, Gunson B, et al. A re-evaluation of the risk factors for the recurrence of primary sclerosing cholangitis in liver allografts. Liver Transpl 2009;15:330.
51. Berstad AE, Aabakken L, Smith HJ, et al. Diagnostic accuracy of magnetic resonance and endoscopic retrograde cholangiography in primary sclerosing cholangitis. Clin Gastroenterol Hepatol 2006;4:514.

Endoscopic Management of Biliary Complications After Liver Transplantation

Karen L. Krok, MD[a], Andrés Cárdenas, MD, MMSc[b,*], Paul J. Thuluvath, MD, FRCP[c]

KEYWORDS

- Liver transplantation • Endoscopy • Biliary complications
- Endoscopic retrograde cholangiography

Biliary tract complications occur in 5% to 25% of patients following liver transplantation (LT).[1–6] These complications include biliary strictures, anastomotic leaks, choledocholithiasis, and biliary casts and can occur after any type of LT, including deceased donor and living-related LT. Because of the small diameter of the anastomotic bile duct, biliary strictures are known to be more common in living-related transplants than in deceased-donor transplants.[7–10] A team approach including hepatologists, endoscopists, transplant surgeons, and interventional radiologists results in the most effective and efficient treatment approach for these patients.

RISK FACTORS FOR BILIARY COMPLICATIONS

There are several known risk factors for the development of biliary complications after LT. Hepatic artery thrombosis can lead to complex hilar strictures as the blood supply to the bile ducts is solely via the hepatic artery. There are several technical factors during surgery that can lead to biliary problems and these include excessive dissection of periductal tissue during procurement, excessive use of electrocautery for biliary duct bleeding control in both donor and recipient, and tension of the duct

[a] Division of Gastroenterology, University of Pennsylvania School of Medicine, 3400 Spruce Street, 3 Ravdin, Philadelphia, PA 19104, USA
[b] GI Unit / Institut Clinic de Malalties Digestives i Metaboliques, University of Barcelona, Hospital Clinic, Villarroel 170, Barcelona 08036, Spain
[c] Center for Liver and Biliary Diseases, Institute for Digestive Health & Liver Disease, Mercy Medical Center, 301 St Paul Place, Baltimore, MD 21202-2165, USA
* Corresponding author.
E-mail address: acardena@clinic.ub.es

Clin Liver Dis 14 (2010) 359–371
doi:10.1016/j.cld.2010.03.008

anastomosis. The donated organ itself can be a risk if it is a donation after cardiac death, if the donor was of an older age, or if there was prolonged cold and warm ischemia time.[11] Pre-LT diagnosis of cytomegalovirus infection also is associated with an increased risk of biliary complications.[12,13]

T-tubes once were placed routinely after an LT for prophylaxis against anastomotic strictures. Their role in the era of endoscopic therapy for strictures is now much less apparent; comparative studies between post-LT patients with and without T-tubes indicate that routine T-tube placement is associated with a higher incidence of biliary complications including bile leaks and cholangitis.[14,15] A recent meta-analysis in more than 1000 patients indicated that those patients without a T-tube had better outcomes compared with those with a T-tube, including fewer episodes of cholangitis and fewer episodes of peritonitis as well as a favorable trend for overall biliary complications. The analysis favored the abandonment of T-tubes in orthotopic LT (OLT).[16]

The type of biliary reconstruction (duct-to-duct choledocho-choledochostomy versus Roux-en-Y choledochojejunostomy) has been suggested as a risk factor for biliary complications. It now is generally agreed that the rate of complications is similar with the Roux-en-Y choledochojejunostomy[2,17] but the duct-to-duct choledocho-choledochostomy has the advantage of easy endoscopic access to the biliary system and preservation of the sphincter of Oddi, which in theory avoids reflux of contents into the bile duct and reduces the risk of cholangitis.[18]

LIVING-DONOR LIVER TRANSPLANTATION AS A RISK FACTOR FOR BILIARY COMPLICATIONS

Living-donor liver transplantation (LDLT) has been associated with a higher rate of bile leaks than in deceased-donor transplantation: 31.8% versus 10.2%, respectively.[19] Factors that are associated significantly with increased biliary leaks are a donor with 3 or more bile ducts, a recipient diagnosis of hepatitis C, and the experience of the transplant center at performing LDLT. Once a center has performed more than 40 LDLTs, the incidence of biliary strictures and biliary leaks decreases significantly. An increased incidence of biliary strictures also is associated with long duration of surgery. Donor age older than 50 and a model for end stage liver disease score greater than 35 are also risk factors for anastomotic strictures in LDLT.[20,21]

The most likely reason for these complications include a relatively smaller duct size, hence a more technically difficult anastomosis, and a higher chance of ischemic injury to the allograft. The anatomic biliary diversity, the more complicated surgical procedure, and if there is a need for multiple reconstructions are contributing factors for the development of biliary complications.[22] Overall, biliary complications occur more frequently in right liver graft recipients than with left liver grafts. In right liver graft recipients with single biliary reconstruction, duct-to-duct anastomosis involving a small-sized duct (<4 mm in diameter) is more of a risk for biliary complications than when a hepatico-jejunostomy is used with these duct sizes.[23] A decreased incidence of biliary complications with a Roux-en-Y reconstruction has been found in some,[19] but not all, studies.[24]

Endoscopic management in LDLT recipients may be quite difficult because of the complex nature of the duct-to-duct reconstruction. Patients will often require frequent endoscopic retrograde cholangiographies (ERCs) with the use of smaller caliber stents (7.0–8.5 Fr). ERC with balloon dilatation is successful in up to 65% of patients. Failure of a primary ERC with dilatation is associated with the appearance of late biliary strictures over 24 weeks from LT and more than 8 weeks between a twofold increase in serum alkaline phosphatase.[25] The relapse rate of strictures is up to 30% and occurs more in patients with shorter duration of stenting; one study found that the duration of stenting in patients with recurrence of strictures was 11.80 $\pm$ 5.03 weeks versus 29.0 $\pm$ 11.6 weeks in the patients who did not have a recurrence of the stricture.[25]

In addition to the recipient, donors also experience biliary complications and should be made aware of this before undergoing donation. In a multicenter study that evaluated the outcome of 393 donors, bile leaks occurred in 36 patients (9%) and most of these patients required a prolonged intensive care unit stay.[26] Biliary complications in donors are seen more often with right lobe donation and the management is the same as described for the recipients.

DIAGNOSTIC APPROACH

Although occasionally patients will have nonspecific symptoms (fever and anorexia), right upper quadrant abdominal pain (especially with bile leaks), pruritus, jaundice, or bile ascites, a biliary complication usually is first suspected in asymptomatic LT recipients who have elevations of serum bilirubin, alkaline phosphatase, and/or gamma-glutamyl transferase (GGT) levels. Absence of pain does not exclude a biliary leak (exposure of the peritoneum and other visceral structures to bile usually results in abdominal pain), as pain may be absent in the transplant setting because of immunosuppression and hepatic denervation in some patients.[9,11,18] The challenge for the transplant team is to differentiate obstructive jaundice from one of the many other causes of cholestasis in patients after LT, ie, acute rejection, chronic rejection, recurrence of the primary disease, fibrosing cholestatic hepatitis C, or drug-induced cholestasis.

When a biliary complication is suspected or there is serologic evidence of cholestasis, the initial evaluation should include a liver ultrasound (US) with a Doppler evaluation of the hepatic vessels. If hepatic artery stenosis or occlusion is suspected by Doppler US, hepatic angiography usually is indicated before continuing with other tests. It is important to remember that an abdominal US may not be sufficiently sensitive (sensitivity 38%–66%) to detect biliary obstruction in the post-LT setting.[27] Thus, the absence of bile duct dilation on US absolutely should not preclude further evaluation with more sensitive techniques in patients in whom there is clinical suspicion of biliary tract complications.

Diagnosis of biliary tract complications after LT is facilitated by the use of noninvasive imaging techniques. Although ERC or percutaneous cholangiography (PTC) remains the gold standard, magnetic resonance cholangiopancreatography (MRCP) is accepted as a reliable and optimal noninvasive technique for detecting biliary complications after LT (sensitivity of 93%–97% and a specificity of 92%–98% compared with ERC as the reference standard).[28–31] An MRCP can provide the endoscopist or interventional radiologist with a map of the reconstructed bile ducts and can be useful especially for obstructions at the hilum or for intrahepatic duct anastomoses; unlike with an ERC, the MRCP has the advantage of demonstrating ducts above and below a stricture (**Fig. 1**). However, an MRCP often will demonstrate some stenosis at the duct-to-duct anastomosis without assessment of severity or significance and has a limited ability to detect biliary sludge and small stones.

In those in whom an invasive approach (ie, ERC or PTC) is required, PTC generally should be reserved for patients in whom ERC was unsuccessful or in patients with a Roux-en-Y choledochojejunostomy. Balloon enteroscopy ERC is now being performed in some centers and may prevent the need for a PTC in those patients with a Roux-en-Y anastomosis.

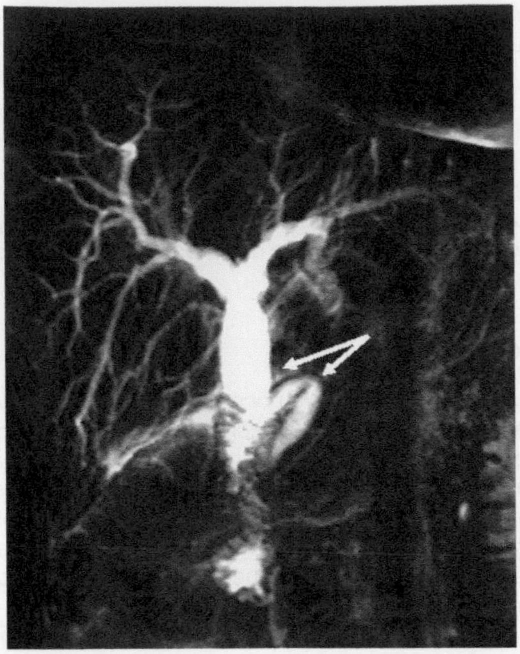

Fig. 1. MRI of a patient after OLT who presented with asymptomatic cholestasis. Note the curved shape of the bile duct and kinking at the distal end (*arrows*).

A liver biopsy is often performed to exclude rejection or recurrent fibrosing cholestatic hepatitis C, although it is generally deferred in patients with biliary dilation or the presence of common bile duct stones because of the risk of causing a bile leak. In these patients, the ERC is performed first and if there is no resolution of the cholestasis, then a liver biopsy is warranted.

ETIOLOGY AND TYPES OF BILIARY STRICTURES

Bile duct strictures occur in 4% to 13% of patients after deceased-donor LT and account for approximately 40% of all biliary complications after LT.[1–6,10,11,32] Higher incidences are found in reports with longer follow-up.[10] The mean time from LT to diagnosis of strictures has been reported to be approximately 2 months.[33] Strictures that occur early after LT are mostly attributable to technical problems, whereas late strictures are mainly attributable to vascular insufficiency and problems with healing and fibrosis.[18,34] A bile leak is an independent risk factor for the development of a stricture and for that reason a bile leak requires emergent endoscopic therapy.[13]

Strictures are classified as anastomotic (AS) or nonanastomotic (NAS), depending on the stricture site; the NAS are often referred to as ischemic strictures and are defined as strictures that occur more than 0.5 cm proximal to the anastomosis. Strictures also can be categorized as early (within the first month of LT) or late (more than 1 month after LT).[33] The clinical significance of this is that the median duration of endoscopic therapy to reach initial success is much longer (up to 2 years) in patients with late-onset strictures.[5,33] For the purpose of this article, we will classify the strictures as AS or NAS, as these 2 types of strictures differ in presentation, outcome, and response to therapy.

Anastomotic Strictures

Up to 80% of biliary strictures are anastomotic, occurring either at the choledocho-choledochostomy or choledochojejunostomy sites.[2,6] Anastomotic strictures typically reflect technical problems at the anastomosis, primarily small bile leaks resulting in a peri-anastomotic fibro-inflammatory response, or ischemia at the end of the bile duct resulting in a fibro-proliferative response. By definition, they are single and short in length, making them suitable for endoscopic intervention (**Fig. 2**).

The characteristic cholangiographic appearance of AS is that of a thin narrowing in the area of the biliary anastomosis (see **Fig. 2**; **Fig. 3**). In some patients, a narrowing of the anastomosis may become evident within the first 1 to 2 months after LT because of postoperative edema and inflammation.[9] This type of narrowing has an excellent response to endoscopic balloon dilation and plastic stent placement; in most patients, it resolves within 3 months and the anastomosis remains patent without further intervention.

Except for the subset of patients with this early narrowing, most patients with AS require ongoing ERC sessions (every 2 to 3 months) with balloon dilation and long-term stenting (for 12 to 24 months). In most cases, an approach using balloon dilation with diameters of 6 to 8 mm and placement of 7.0- to 11.5-Fr plastic stents is more effective than balloon dilation alone.[35] Stents should be exchanged at 3-month intervals to avoid stent occlusion and the precipitation of bacterial cholangitis. Most patients require several endoscopic interventions (mean of 3 to 5) with long-term success rates in the range of 70% to 100%.[3,9,32,33,35–38] The placement of a progressively increasing number of as well as diameter stents with each subsequent ERC has been shown to be a successful method of treating AS (**Fig. 4**).[37] In an illustrative study, patients who developed biliary strictures after LT and who initially were treated endoscopically with balloon dilation and plastic stents had a recurrence rate of 18% with a mean time to recurrence of 110 days.[39]

There is some clinical experience in temporary placement of a covered self-expanding metal stent to reduce the need for repeated stent exchanges, but data are limited.[40] The difficulty with the uncovered metallic self-expandable stent is that there is an inevitable reactive hyperplasia that can be accompanied by secondary stone formation above the stent and there may be a challenge in removing the stent once

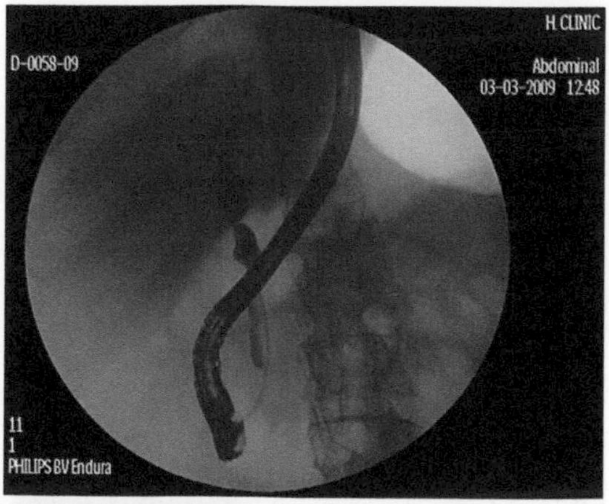

Fig. 2. Anastomotic stricture in a patient after OLT. Note the short segment narrowed area and the biliary dilation.

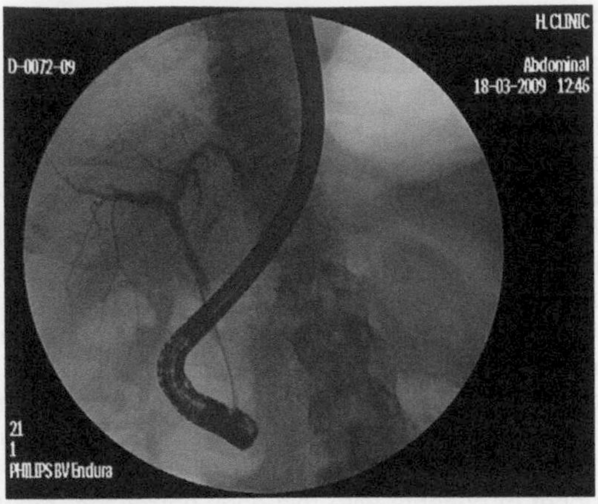

Fig. 3. An astomotic stricture in another patient after OLT. Note the slightly longer segment with thin narrowing with any significant biliary dilation.

it has been in place for 6 to 9 months.[41] Fully covered stents, by contrast, almost always are able to be removed endoscopically, as they do not embed into the surrounding tissue. The data on this type of stent are limited and one article reported the stents caused strictures in the bile duct mainly secondary to the anchoring point in the distal proximal end.[42] Additionally, they may occlude secondary branch ducts, limiting their use in patients with right-lobe live-donor transplants. More data are needed to consider the routine use of covered stents in AS after OLT.

Because of these high rates of success, endoscopic management should be considered the first choice before considering percutaneous interventions or surgical repair in patients with duct-to-duct anastomosis. In patients with Roux-en-Y choledochojejunostomy, management with balloon enteroscopy ERC or PTC and dilation followed by placement of a percutaneous transhepatic catheter is often necessary. Surgical intervention (usually a repair or conversion to a Roux-en-Y choledochojejunostomy) is required when the ERC or PTC fails to adequately treat AS. An advantage of surgery is that it eliminates the need for multiple procedures.

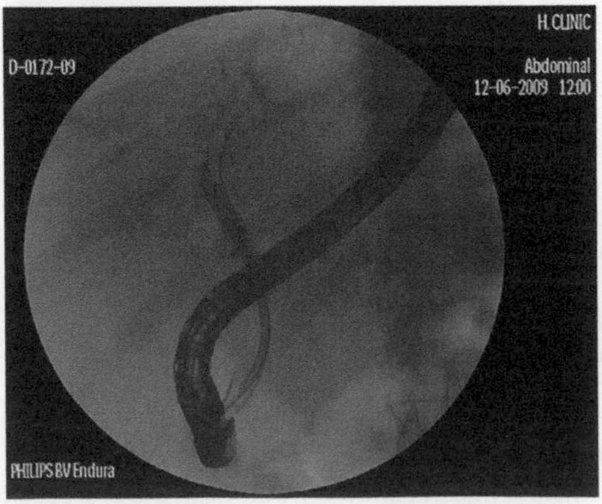

Fig. 4. Two plastic stents placed side by side after dilation of an anastomotic stricture.

Nonanastomotic Strictures

Nonanastomotic strictures (or ischemic strictures) result mainly from hepatic artery thrombosis, increased cold ischemia time, or ABO blood-type incompatibility. There is felt to be peribiliary arteriolar endothelial injury resulting in irreversible microvascular thrombosis.[10] Less commonly these strictures can be caused by recurrence of the underlying disease such as primary sclerosing cholangitis. They account for 10.0% to 25.0% of all stricture complications after LT, with an incidence in the range of 0.5% to 10.0%.[1–6]

True ischemic strictures occur more than 0.5 cm proximal to the anastomosis and often involve the hilum and multiple separate obstructions at the level of the sectoral or segmental branch ducts. This can lead to a cholangiographic appearance that resembles primary sclerosing cholangitis. Biliary sludge can accumulate proximal to the strictures leading to the formation of casts.[17] NAS tend to occur earlier than AS, with a mean time to stricture development of 3 to 6 months.[6,11]

NAS are generally more difficult to treat than AS and include multiple episodes of cholangitis and hospitalizations. Endoscopic therapy of NAS typically consists of 4- to 6-mm balloon dilation (compared with 6 to 8 mm for AS) followed by sphincterotomy, and placement of a 10.0- to 11.5-Fr plastic stent with replacement every 3 months, similar to the management of AS.[5] The more aggressive approach with the placement of a progressively increasing number of as well as diameter stents with each subsequent ERC has been shown to be a successful method of treating NAS.[37] However, time to response with NAS is more prolonged than with AS and patients with NAS require twice the number of interventions as patients with AS. The median time to resolution of the stricture on average is 185 days for NAS versus 67 days for AS.[11]

The outcomes of NAS are not as favorable as AS. The 5-year graft survival rate is 73% in patients with NAS, which is significantly lower than in matched controls without strictures.[43] Only 50% to 75% of patients have a long-term response with endoscopic therapy with dilation and stent placement.[5,9,11,44,45] Furthermore, up to 30% to 50% of patients undergo retransplantation or die as a consequence of this complication despite endoscopic therapy.[5,6,14,18] As a general rule, ischemic events that lead to diffuse intrahepatic bile duct strictures are associated with poor graft survival and will require retransplantation in suitable candidates.

Surgical revision may ultimately be required in patients with strictures that are refractory to endoscopic or percutaneous treatment. A Roux-en-Y choledochojejunostomy is usually performed in patients with duct-to-duct anastomosis. In those who already have a Roux-en-Y anastomosis, a revision may be required by repositioning the bile duct of the graft to a more highly vascularized area.

BILIARY LEAKS

The incidence of biliary leaks after LT ranges between 2% and 25%.[1–6,46,47] Bile leaks can occur from the anastomosis, the cystic duct remnant, the T-tube tract, or (in the case of living donor LT) from the cut surface of the liver. Many bile leaks can be resolved nonoperatively with early intervention.[1–6,46]

When there is a low suspicion of a biliary leak, a radionucleotide scan has reasonable accuracy at noninvasive detection of a bile leak.[48] ERC, though, is the gold standard diagnostic method and should be performed in all patients when there is a high suspicion for biliary leaks (**Fig. 5**). Treatment for biliary leaks consists of placement of either an endoscopic stent and/or a percutaneous stent/drain. If there is an associated stricture, then both the leak and the stricture need to be bridged by the stent. Stent

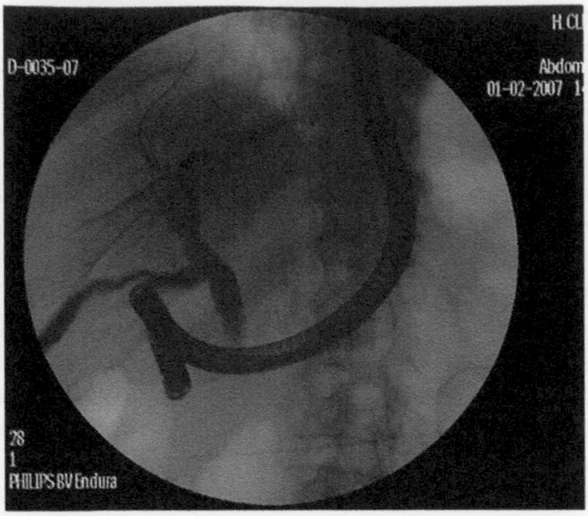

Fig. 5. Significant bile leak after liver transplantation.

placement can result in up to 88% resolution of biliary leaks. Resolution of the leak occurs typically within 5 weeks but the patient's symptoms will resolve within days of stent insertion.[36] In contrast to post-cholecystectomy leaks, where the stent can be removed in 4 to 6 weeks, in post-LT leaks the stent should be left in place for approximately 2 to 3 months because of problems with delayed healing that may arise as a result of immunosuppression.[11] In cases where a T-tube is in place, small anastomotic leaks can be diagnosed with a T-tube cholangiogram and can be managed by leaving the tube open without further intervention. Instead of the transpapillary stent, a nasobiliary tube can be inserted. An advantage of the nasobiliary tubes is that they permit cholangiographic follow-up without the need for further endoscopies[49]; however, they are often poorly tolerated and also divert bile away from the intestine, thereby decreasing the bioavailability of certain drugs.

Roux-en-Y choledochojejunostomy anastomotic leaks are less common. A suspected bile leak in such patients can be diagnosed with a hepatobiliary imino-diacetic acid scan if patients do not have a drainage catheter in place. Standard ERC is often not feasible because of anatomic difficulties in reaching the biliary anastomosis. Management is usually performed with percutaneous internal-external drainage. Bile leaks in patients with Roux-en-Y anatomy more often require surgical management.

Bile leaks have been classified as early or late depending on if they occur before or after 1 month from the LT. Early bile leaks usually occur at the anastomotic site and are often related to technical issues, not to the type of biliary reconstruction. Factors that predispose grafts to early bile leaks include lack of perfusion from the hepatic artery and other technical reasons. Bile leaks are suspected in patients with peritonitis or fluid collections seen on imaging tests. Late bile duct leaks usually are related to the removal of the T-tube, resulting from delay in T-tube tract maturation as a result of immunosuppression. A bile leak should be suspected in patients who develop pain when the T-tube is removed. A relatively higher proportion of patients with late bile leaks later present with biliary strictures than do those with early leaks; the transplant team should have a high clinical suspicion for a biliary stricture in these patients if the alkaline phosphatase, total bilirubin, or GGT increase.

Bilomas occur because of bile duct rupture and extravasation of bile into the hepatic parenchyma or the abdominal cavity. Most post-LT bilomas occur in the perihepatic area. Large bilomas not communicating with the bile ducts should be treated with percutaneous drainage and antibiotics. Surgery is indicated only when the bile leak cannot be controlled effectively with endoscopic stenting.

BILIARY STONES, SLUDGE, AND CASTS

Biliary filling defects occur in approximately 5% of patients after liver transplantation.[47] These filling defects can be caused by gallstones, sludge, debris, blood clots, casts, or migrated stents; as many as 70% of such defects are caused by stones.[5,9] Management is similar to the nontransplant setting (with sphincterotomy and balloon or basket extraction) with the caveat that in the presence of immunosuppressive agents, patients can have a rapid clinical decline. Patients can present with recurrent attacks of cholangitis, sepsis, or pancreatitis or may simply have cholestasis without associated pain.

Biliary strictures, bacterial infections, and obstructions can predispose a patient to the formation of biliary stones or sludge. In addition, a history of hepatic artery thrombosis and a prolonged cold ischemia time are associated with debris formation.[47]

Stones

Stones usually form above a stricture or stenosis. Cyclosporine is known to promote supersaturation of bile and may contribute to the formation of biliary stones. In one series, stones appeared a median of 19 months after LT; interestingly, following stone extraction there is a 17% recurrence rate within a median of 6 months.[44] In most cases (59% to 66%), a single ERC session with biliary sphincterotomy and balloon or basket extraction is sufficient to clear the duct of distal stones[44]; however, 2 sessions may be required in 24% of patients and 3 or more sessions may be required in 17% of patients.[44] Advanced ERC techniques, such as intraductal lithotripsy or direct choledochoscopy may be required.

Casts

Biliary casts develop in 18% of LT recipients. Cast development is associated with acute cellular rejection, ischemia, infection, and biliary obstruction. Bile duct casts most commonly develop in the setting of ischemia (for example, hepatic artery thrombosis) when there is diffuse stricturing of the hilum.[17] Clearance of casts is successful in 60% of patients using endoscopic and percutaneous methods.[17] Various combinations of sphincterotomy, balloon and basket extraction, stent placement, and lithotripsy are often necessary. Patients with Roux-en-Y choledochojejunostomy should be treated initially with a percutaneous method. Surgery is offered only when percutaneous and endoscopic methods are not successful.

Biliary cast syndrome is the presence of multiple casts and refers to the development of a hardened, dark material within the biliary system that takes the physical shape of the bile ducts. The disorder occurs in 2.5% to 18.0% of liver transplant recipients[27,47,50] and is associated with increased morbidity, mortality, and incidence of rejection.[27] Typically it occurs within the first year after transplantation. Analysis of the casts has shown that bilirubin is the primary element along with collagen, bile acid, and cholesterol.[51–53] The true pathogenesis of biliary cast syndrome is unknown but it is believed that ischemic factors and biliary strictures play an important role in its development. Another risk factor is an increase in warm ischemia time.[27] In one study, patients with biliary cast syndrome had a warm ischemia time of 48 minutes compared with only 40 minutes in patients without biliary cast syndrome (P<.0001).[54] Several endoscopic approaches have been described with variable success and often multiple procedures are required. Unfortunately it has been reported that up to 22% of patients with biliary cast syndrome will require retransplantation.

SPHINCTER OF ODDI DYSFUNCTION

The sphincter of Oddi is a muscular structure that encompasses the confluence of the distal common bile duct and the pancreatic duct as they penetrate the wall of the duodenum. The term sphincter of Oddi dysfunction (SOD) has been used to describe a clinical syndrome of biliary or pancreatic obstruction related to mechanical or functional abnormalities of the sphincter of Oddi. It is postulated that in the posttransplant setting, denervation of the common bile duct in the ampullary region (secondary to surgical intervention) may lead to the development of a hypertonic sphincter causing SOD. SOD has been described in 2% to 7% of patients who undergo LT.[1,45]

SOD should be suspected in patients with cholestasis and a uniformly dilated bile duct without filling defects; abdominal pain may not be present. SOD also may contribute to pancreatitis and should be considered in the differential when a cause for the pancreatitis has not been found. As for SOD in the nontransplant setting, the risk of pancreatitis after an ERC is high and so temporary prophylactic pancreatic stents after sphincterotomy should be placed if possible to avoid this risk.

SUMMARY

Biliary complications are common in recipients of deceased-donor and live-donor liver transplants and can occur in up to 9% of donors as well. These complications include biliary strictures, bile leaks, biliary obstruction (with stones, sludge, or casts), and sphincter of Oddi dysfunction. Given the frequency of these complications and the risk for significant impact on the transplanted organ, the transplant team needs to work closely with endoscopists and interventional radiologists to treat these lesions in an expedient manner.

REFERENCES

1. Stratta RJ, Wood RP, Langnas AN, et al. Diagnosis and treatment of biliary tract complications after orthotopic liver transplantation. Surgery 1989;106(4):675–83 [discussion: 683–4].
2. Greif F, Bronsther OL, Van Thiel DH, et al. The incidence, timing, and management of biliary tract complications after orthotopic liver transplantation. Ann Surg 1994;219(1):40–5.
3. Rerknimitr R, Sherman S, Fogel EL, et al. Biliary tract complications after orthotopic liver transplantation with choledochocholedochostomy anastomosis: endoscopic findings and results of therapy. Gastrointest Endosc 2002;55(2):224–31.
4. Pfau PR, Kochman ML, Lewis JD, et al. Endoscopic management of postoperative biliary complications in orthotopic liver transplantation. Gastrointest Endosc 2000;52(1):55–63.
5. Thuluvath PJ, Atassi T, Lee J. An endoscopic approach to biliary complications following orthotopic liver transplantation. Liver Int 2003;23(3):156–62.
6. Thethy S, Thomson B, Pleass H, et al. Management of biliary tract complications after orthotopic liver transplantation. Clin Transplant 2004;18(6):647–53.
7. Trotter JF, Wachs M, Everson GT, et al. Adult-to-adult transplantation of the right hepatic lobe from a living donor. N Engl J Med 2002;346(14):1074–82.
8. Busuttil RW, Farmer DG, Yersiz H, et al. Analysis of long-term outcomes of 3200 liver transplantations over two decades: a single-center experience. Ann Surg 2005;241(6):905–16 [discussion: 916–8].
9. Verdonk RC, Buis CI, Porte RJ, et al. Anastomotic biliary strictures after liver transplantation: causes and consequences. Liver Transpl 2006;12(5):726–35.

10. Koneru B, Sterling MJ, Bahramipour PF. Bile duct strictures after liver transplantation: a changing landscape of the Achilles' heel. Liver Transpl 2006;12(5):702–4.
11. Thuluvath PJ, Pfau PR, Kimmey MB, et al. Biliary complications after liver transplantation: the role of Endoscopy. Endoscopy 2005;37(9):857–63.
12. Maheshwari A, Maley W, Li Z, et al. Biliary complications and outcomes of liver transplantation from donors after cardiac death. Liver Transpl 2007;13(12): 1645–53.
13. Welling TH, Heidt DG, Englesbe MJ, et al. Biliary complications following liver transplantation in the model for end-stage liver disease era: effect of donor, recipient, and technical factors. Liver Transpl 2008;14(1):73–80.
14. Scatton O, Meunier B, Cherqui D, et al. Randomized trial of choledochocholedochostomy with or without a T tube in orthotopic liver transplantation. Ann Surg 2001;233(3):432–7.
15. Vougas V, Rela M, Gane E, et al. A prospective randomised trial of bile duct reconstruction at liver transplantation: T tube or no T tube? Transpl Int 1996; 9(4):392–5.
16. Sotiropoulos GC, Sgourakis G, Radtke A, et al. Orthotopic liver transplantation: T-tube or no T-tube? Systematic review and meta-analysis of results. Transplantation 2009;87(11):1672–80.
17. Davidson BR, Rai R, Kurzawinski TR, et al. Prospective randomized trial of end-to-end versus side-to-side biliary reconstruction after orthotopic liver transplantation. Br J Surg 1999;86(4):447–52.
18. Pascher A, Neuhaus P. Biliary complications after deceased-donor orthotopic liver transplantation. J Hepatobiliary Pancreat Surg 2006;13(6):487–96.
19. Freise CE, Gillespie BW, Koffron AJ, et al. Recipient morbidity after living and deceased donor liver transplantation: findings from the A2ALL Retrospective Cohort Study. Am J Transplant 2008;8(12):2569–79.
20. Shah SA, Grant DR, McGilvray ID, et al. Biliary strictures in 130 consecutive right lobe living donor liver transplant recipients: results of a Western center. Am J Transplant 2007;7(1):161–7.
21. Liu CL, Lo CM, Chan SC, et al. Safety of duct-to-duct biliary reconstruction in right-lobe live-donor liver transplantation without biliary drainage. Transplantation 2004;77(5):726–32.
22. Gondolesi GE, Varotti G, Florman SS, et al. Biliary complications in 96 consecutive right lobe living donor transplant recipients. Transplantation 2004;77(12): 1842–8.
23. Hwang S, Lee SG, Sung KB, et al. Long-term incidence, risk factors, and management of biliary complications after adult living donor liver transplantation. Liver Transpl 2006;12(5):831–8.
24. Soejima Y, Taketomi A, Yoshizumi T, et al. Biliary strictures in living donor liver transplantation: incidence, management, and technical evolution. Liver Transpl 2006;12(6):979–86.
25. Seo JK, Ryu JK, Lee SH, et al. Endoscopic treatment for biliary stricture after adult living donor liver transplantation. Liver Transpl 2009;15(4):369–80.
26. Ghobrial RM, Freise CE, Trotter JF, et al. Donor morbidity after living donation for liver transplantation. Gastroenterology 2008;135:468.
27. Sharma S, Gurakar A, Jabbour N. Biliary strictures following liver transplantation: past, present and preventive strategies. Liver Transpl 2008;14(6):759–69.
28. Beltran MM, Marugan RB, Oton E, et al. Accuracy of magnetic resonance cholangiography in the evaluation of late biliary complications after orthotopic liver transplantation. Transplant Proc 2005;37(9):3924–5.

29. Linhares MM, Gonzalez AM, Goldman SM, et al. Magnetic resonance cholangiography in the diagnosis of biliary complications after orthotopic liver transplantation. Transplant Proc 2004;36(4):947–8.
30. Boraschi P, Braccini G, Gigoni R, et al. Detection of biliary complications after orthotopic liver transplantation with MR cholangiography. Magn Reson Imaging 2001;19(8):1097–105.
31. Novellas S, Caramella T, Fournol M, et al. MR cholangiopancreatography features of the biliary tree after liver transplantation. AJR Am J Roentgenol 2008;191(1):221–7.
32. Graziadei IW, Schwaighofer H, Koch R, et al. Long-term outcome of endoscopic treatment of biliary strictures after liver transplantation. Liver Transpl 2006;12(5):718–25.
33. Pasha SF, Harrison ME, Das A, et al. Endoscopic treatment of anastomotic biliary strictures after deceased donor liver transplantation: outcomes after maximal stent therapy. Gastrointest Endosc 2007;66(1):44–51.
34. Testa G, Malago M, Broelseh CE. Complications of biliary tract in liver transplantation. World J Surg 2001;25(10):1296–9.
35. Zoepf T, Maldonado-Lopez EJ, Hilgard P, et al. Balloon dilatation vs. balloon dilatation plus bile duct endoprostheses for treatment of anastomotic biliary strictures after liver transplantation. Liver Transpl 2006;12(1):88–94.
36. Morelli J, Mulcahy HE, Willner IR, et al. Long-term outcomes for patients with post-liver transplant anastomotic biliary strictures treated by endoscopic stent placement. Gastrointest Endosc 2003;58(3):374–9.
37. Holt AP, Thorburn D, Mirza D, et al. A prospective study of standardized nonsurgical therapy in the management of biliary anastomotic strictures complicating liver transplantation. Transplantation 2007;84(7):857–63.
38. Kulaksiz H, Weiss KH, Gotthardt D, et al. Is stenting necessary after balloon dilation of post-transplantation biliary strictures? Results of a prospective comparative study. Endoscopy 2008;40(9):746–51.
39. Alazmi WM, Fogel EL, Watkins JL, et al. Recurrence rate of anastomotic biliary strictures in patients who have had previous successful endoscopic therapy for anastomotic narrowing after orthotopic liver transplantation. Endoscopy 2006;38(6):571–4.
40. Kahaleh M, Behm B, Clarke BW, et al. Temporary placement of covered self-expandable metal stents in benign biliary strictures: a new paradigm? (with video). Gastrointest Endosc 2008;67(3):446–54.
41. Larghi A, Tringali A, Lecca PG, et al. Management of hilar biliary strictures. Am J Gastroenterol 2008;103(2):458–73.
42. Wang AY, Ellen K, Berg CL, et al. Fully covered self-expandable metallic stents in the management of complex biliary leaks: preliminary data—a case series. Endoscopy 2009;41(9):781–6.
43. Verdonk RC, Buis CI, van der Jagt EJ, et al. Nonanastomotic biliary strictures after liver transplantation, part 2: management, outcome, and risk factors for disease progression. Liver Transpl 2007;13(5):725–32.
44. Park JS, Kim MH, Lee SK, et al. Efficacy of endoscopic and percutaneous treatments for biliary complications after cadaveric and living donor liver transplantation. Gastrointest Endosc 2003;57(1):78–85.
45. Sawyer RG, Punch JD. Incidence and management of biliary complications after 291 liver transplants following the introduction of transcystic stenting. Transplantation 1998;66(9):1201–7.
46. Scanga AE, Kowdley KV. Management of biliary complications following orthotopic liver transplantation. Curr Gastroenterol Rep 2007;9(1):31–8.

47. Sheng R, Sammon JK, Zajko AB, et al. Bile leak after hepatic transplantation: cholangiographic features, prevalence, and clinical outcome. Radiology 1994; 192(2):413–6.
48. Roca I, Ciofetta G. Hepatobiliary scintigraphy in current pediatric practice. Q J Nucl Med 1998;42(2):113–8.
49. Saab S, Martin P, Soliman GY, et al. Endoscopic management of biliary leaks after T-tube removal in liver transplant recipients: nasobiliary drainage versus biliary stenting. Liver Transpl 2000;6(5):627–32.
50. Barton P, Maier A, Steininger R, et al. Biliary sludge after liver transplantation: 1. Imaging findings and efficacy of various imaging procedures. AJR Am J Roentgenol 1995;164(4):859–64.
51. Waldram R, Williams R, Calne RY. Bile composition and bile cast formation after transplantation of the liver in man. Transplantation 1975;19(5):382–7.
52. Canete JJ, Aidlen JT, Uknis ME, et al. Images of interest. Hepatobiliary and pancreatic: biliary cast syndrome. J Gastroenterol Hepatol 2005;20(5):791.
53. Shah JN, Haigh WG, Lee SP, et al. Biliary casts after orthotopic liver transplantation: clinical factors, treatment, biochemical analysis. Am J Gastroenterol 2003; 98(8):1861–7.
54. Gor NV, Levy RM, Ahn J, et al. Biliary cast syndrome following liver transplantation: predictive factors and clinical outcomes. Liver Transpl 2008;14:1466–72.

Index

Note: Page numbers of article titles are in **boldface** type.

Clin Liver Dis 14 (2010) 373–380
doi:10.1016/S1089-3261(10)00026-7

F

G

H

P

R

S

Printed and bound by CPI Group (UK) Ltd, Croydon, CR0 4YY
14/10/2024
01773702-0002